The PERIPATETIC DIABETIC

Also by June Biermann and Barbara Toohey
The Diabetic's Book: All Your Questions Answered
The Woman's Holistic Headache Relief Book
The Diabetic's Sports & Exercise Book
The Diabetes Question & Answer Book
The Diabetic's Total Health Book

Under the name Margaret Bennett
Biking for Grownups
Cross-Country Skiing for the Fun of It
How to Ski Just a Little Bit
The Peripatetic Diabetic
Dr. Owl's Problem
From Baedeker to Worse
Alice in Womanland

The
PERIPATETIC
DIABETIC

June Biermann   Barbara Toohey

JEREMY P. TARCHER, INC.
Los Angeles
Distributed by Houghton Mifflin Company
Boston

Library of Congress Cataloging in Publication Data

Biermann, June.
  The peripatetic diabetic.

  Previously issued under the authors' joint pseudonym: Margaret Bennett.
  Originally published: New York: Hawthorn Books, 1969.
  Includes index.
  1. Diabetes. 2. Diabetes—Diet therapy. I. Toohey, Barbara. II. Title.
RC660.B48 1984   616.4'62   83-24336
ISBN 0–87477–309–1
ISBN 0–87477–308–3 (ppbk.)

Requests for such permissions should be addressed to:
Jeremy P. Tarcher, Inc.
9110 Sunset Blvd.
Los Angeles, CA 90069

Manufactured in the United States of America
S 10 9 8 7 6 5 4 3 2 1

To Banting and Best,
the discoverers of insulin,
and to the Juvenile Diabetes Foundation,
which may someday eliminate
the necessity for their discovery

ACKNOWLEDGMENTS

We are grateful for permission to quote from the following: *Brave New World* by Aldous Huxley (Harper & Row, Publishers); *Diabetes in the News*, January-February-March 1968 Edition, Volume 7, No. 1; "Équivalences à l'Étranger des Diverses Marques d'Insulines Vendues en France" and "Équivalences à l'Étrangerger des Diverses Marques de Produits Antidiabétiques Oraux Vendues en France" by the Association Française des Diabétiques; "Explanation of the Food-Exchange System" and "Expanded Exchange Lists" by Mrs. T. W. Vaught; Tom Gess in *The Diabetic; A Guide for the Diabetic*, 1966 Edition (Eli Lilly and Company); "Holidays" by Iris Holland Rogers (The British Diabetic Association); *How to Live with Diabetes* by Henry Dolger, M.D., and Bernard Seeman (W. W. Norton & Company, Inc.); "Lament for Prometheus Bound" (*Gourmet*, March 1962); *Playing for Life* by William F. Talbert and John S. Sharnik (Little, Brown and Company); "Wouldn't It Be Easier If I Just Wore a Sign on My Back?" by Joyce Lubold (*Publisher's Weekly*, March 21, 1966).

We are also grateful to Dr. Merritt H. Stiles and Dr. Peter R. Richards for allowing us to quote them.

CONTENTS

INTRODUCTION:
THE SAME OLD CHANGES

In June's reading in Oriental philosophy, she's come to admire Buddhism particularly. She likes its tenets of joy, friendliness, compassion, and equanimity; its meditative aspects (calming and stress reduction are always good for diabetes control); and its doctrine of peace and tolerance. The Buddha has also given us one of our favorite and truest quotes: "The only constant is change."

Nowhere is the constancy of change more evident than in diabetes. It's been sixteen years since the original edition of *The Peripatetic Diabetic* was published, eighteen years since June was diagnosed diabetic. That doesn't seem like a terribly long time, and yet during that period so many changes have taken place in diabetes that it almost seems as though it's a whole new disease. And we've changed. We both feel we're whole new people. In the physical sense, it's true that we literally are renewed since every cell in the body is replaced every twelve years or so. But more than that, our attitudes and lives have changed to such an extent that in rereading the original book, we occasionally have trouble recognizing ourselves.

We especially have trouble recognizing and remembering our collaborative alter ego, Margaret Bennett, under whose auspices *The Peripatetic Diabetic* was written sixteen years ago. She was only a source of confusion, so we've gotten rid of her. We aren't even sure now why we used a pseudonym in the first place.

We also thought of rubbing out the title, which was conceived— perhaps ill conceived—by a perspicacious editor. But we decided against it. Since, after sixteen years, we've finally learned how to spell it, we figured it would be a waste to give it up now.

When we started work on this new edition we planned to go

through the original book and take out errors of fact (for example: disposable syringes are now made by Becton-Dickinson and Monoject, not Becton-Dickinson and Johnson and Johnson; U-80 insulin is no longer available; the current estimate of the number of diabetics is 12 million; and truffles now cost $38.00 an ounce instead of $3.00 an ounce) as well as errors in our thinking (diabetics who are underweight can lap up as much fat as they like). Then we decided that wouldn't be right. It would be like taking something written before Columbus and removing all references to a flat Earth, or like rewriting *Little Women* to have Meg, Jo, Beth, and Amy zipping around in jet planes. Now is now and then was then. June hasn't touched a half inch of Tes-Tape in six years, but in those days her life was festooned with it. So be it. We'll let it stand.

Another reason we've let the original stand as written is that although we believe the Buddha was right about change, we also agree with the French: *Plus ça change, plus c'est la même chose* ("The more it changes, the more it's the same thing"). Diabetes when first diagnosed is still a heavy hit to the diaphragm that knocks the wind out of you and out of your sails. You're still scared, still confused, still certain that the good life is over. So many people have told us, "*The Peripatetic Diabetic* is *my* story; I could have written it; I feel exactly the way June did," that we know the feelings are universal. June is Everydiabetic. Every diabetic is Everydiabetic, and every diabetic can be peripatetic—meaning to get around in every sense of the word.

Later on, in *The Peripatetic Diabetic II*, we'll straighten out the facts and bring you into the contemporary world. But first, the unvarnished truth. First we'll present the original book with all of its alarums and confusions exactly as it was written—and lived.

June Biermann
Barbara Toohey
The Sugarfree Center
P.O. Box 114
Van Nuys, CA 91408
1984

Part One

THE PERIPATETIC DIABETIC

Chapter 1

HOW GREEN
WAS MY TES-TAPE

Along with the many technical writings I've read on diabetes, I've also looked over a few "inspirational" articles by diabetics for diabetics. These usually strum a saccharine note of maudlin sentiment, such as, "Now that I have diabetes I am able to enjoy sunsets and the laughter of little children more." Unladylike expletive!

My enjoyment of sunsets and children's laughter is not dependent upon diabetes. And I resent the tacit suggestion that as a diabetic I must savor each golden moment because it may be my last.

I'm convinced that I will probably live as long with diabetes as I could have without it, for the simple reason that it has caused me to take better care of myself than I would have otherwise. In fact, it's possible that the health regime I adhere to may even prevent my falling victim to something far more serious than diabetes and may extend my allotment of sunsets and children's laughter beyond what it normally would have been.

Still, with no Pollyannics about it, I have to admit that since developing diabetes, I *am* enjoying life more. Not only have I not cut back on any of my old normal activities, but I now do more rather than less than I did before. I don't know why this has come about. It may be that I would have taken up these new activities and interests anyway. Or it may be that having diabetes has made me try new things just to prove to myself that I could do them, to prove that I wasn't handicapped in any way. But though I can't explain all the why's of this upswing in my life, I do have a very accurate picture of how I was able to carry it off. . . .

3

"Are you still sickeningly healthy?" Barbara inquired as I passed her desk in the periodicals room of the library on the way to my office.

I was feeling thoroughly disgruntled. It had been two and a half years since my last "annual checkup," and when I finally forced myself to call my health service it took me six weeks to get an appointment. Then when the day finally rolled around I had to take time off from work, negotiate the freeway to downtown Los Angeles, and wait over an hour to see the doctor. All this for an examination that took only thirty minutes and to me appeared so cursory that it couldn't have uncovered a raging case of chicken pox.

Since I dismissed this unhappy interlude from my mind as quickly as possible, I was more than surprised fourteen days later to receive a call from the health service. "You'll have to come down again," the girl said, "because one of your laboratory tests needs to be repeated." She could not or would not or wasn't allowed to tell me which test needed to be taken over or why. I was more disgusted than ever. I assumed they had made some stupid blunder and I was having to pay for it out of my own time and inconvenience.

With that telephone call I again became a reluctant participant in the most popular and prevalent pastime of the modern world —the waiting game. Wait a week until the next appointment to find out why a test needed to be taken over. Sugar in the urine, they said. Nothing definite, of course. No need to worry. The test often comes out like this and it doesn't mean a thing. Have to take a blood sugar test to know for sure. Wait four days and then for three days eat the high carbohydrate breakfast diet (1 cup orange juice, 1 cup cornflakes, 1 glass milk with 1 tablespoon sugar in it, 1 egg, 2 pieces of toast with 2 tablespoons jam, and coffee) required for a postprandial blood sugar test. Come back to the office for the blood test. Wait four days for the test to be analyzed. Wait for a call from the doctor to come down for the results. Wait a little more in the doctor's waiting room before going in to see him for the verdict.

I wouldn't have minded playing the waiting game so much if I had been able to quit winners. But I lost and lost heavily.

On the memorable occasion of St. Patrick's Day I was given the official results: 440 blood sugar (normal is between 80 and 110) and a definite diagnosis of diabetes. On the way home I stopped at the pharmacy and purchased my first roll of the diabetic serpentine which was to festoon my future life—Tes-Tape, the chemically treated tape which registers sugar in the urine by turning from yellow to green. And when I got home and made my first urine test, my Tes-Tape was so green that, as Barbara said, I could have pinned it to my lapel and worn it in honor of the holiday. I was in no mood for her gallows humor. My mind was churning like a washing machine over what I'd been told.

Diabetes. What was it, anyway? All I knew was that it had something to do with sugar. I had always thought it was brought on by eating too many sweets. It struck me as particularly odd, then, that I should get it, because I had never really cared for candy, rich desserts, hot fudge sundaes, and the like. They had always made my eyes feel as if they were burning and I had avoided them. At any rate, I thought that diabetics couldn't eat sugar, and I decided they couldn't eat much of anything else, either, judging by the 1,800-calorie diabetic exchange list diet the doctor had given me along with my plastic beginner's kit of Orinase, an oral hypoglycemic agent—in other words, the pills that help lower the blood sugar of some diabetics.

Diabetes was, I dimly remembered, an old, established disease that had been around for a long time, not one of those Johnny-come-lately maladies that clever pathologists have just recently isolated and distributed to the general public. Also, it had probably been in *me* for a while, too. I began to sort through my mental files to see if I had had any clue that something might be amiss. And I discovered quite a few retrospectively obvious symptoms which I had ignored or blamed on some other cause, mainly my mind.

Like every other modern American woman, I have been brainwashed into believing that whenever anything is wrong with me it is strictly psychogenic. There have been so many books and articles about neurotic women—especially middle-aged neurotic women—and their imaginary maladies that most of us hesitate to go to the doctor with any complaint at all. One of my friends at the college once went around with a couple of cracked ribs for a month and a half, because she was embarrassed to show up at the doctor's office with vague complaints of "pains in the back." She was certain that after looking her over he would condescendingly tell her that there was nothing really wrong with her and that she should go home and take it easy. He would then slip her a prescription for tranquilizers and nudge her out the door to make room for someone really sick.

Of course, it wasn't too illogical of me to think that my symptoms were all in my mind, because many of them took the form of mental disorders. For a year or so I had had insomnia, lying awake for seeming eternities, especially in the pre-dawn hours, my whole system feeling clenched. On top of that, for days at a time I would fall victim to deep feelings of depression, including periods when all I felt like doing was just sitting and letting tears race down my face. I attributed these neurotic symptoms to a problem of lack of communication with our book editor and to the stresses of writing a book while also holding down a full-time job. After all, Barbara, who is generally 99 and 44/100 percent manic, was having spells of melancholia herself. Probably, I now realize, since we were working together so much of the time, she was just catching my neurosis by osmosis. Anyway, my depressions were far more severe and much more regular than hers.

My symptoms weren't all mental, though. I started having to get up in the middle of the night to go to the bathroom, but this I shrugged off as a result of the insomnia and possibly of getting older. I also began to pick up all the little sicknesses that were going around. This was very odd for me, and I think now that it's what ultimately drove me into the doctor's office for a physical examination. I had never (well, hardly ever) been sick. In the eighteen years I had worked for the Los Angeles City Schools I had been out on sick leave only two days. The first was when the karate chop of the Asian flu got through even my seemingly impenetrable resistance, and the second—I will confess, since this is an extremely honest book—was a hangover.

Not only was I always well, but I was completely unsympathetic and intolerant of sickness in others. When fellow woıkers called into the library to say they were sick with a cold, I would archly inform them that colds are a substitute for crying.

Then suddenly, inexplicably, I began to get sore throats that blossomed into full-blown colds and left lingering laryngitis, as they hung on and on and on. The first of these I remember having while on a tour of Japan in the summer of 1966, and I had just recovered from a San Francisco-trip-induced cold when I had the initial physical examination that eventually spelled out diabetes. No, I had not been myself for some time, and now that I knew I had diabetes, it looked as if I was never going to be myself again.

Although I know now that there are over 2,600,000 discovered diabetics in the country, at that moment I felt I was the only one in the world. There had been no diabetics in my family and I didn't know any diabetics personally. At least, I didn't know I knew any. I later found out there were several among my acquaintances, but they just didn't talk about it. Diabetics, I find, are strange that way. Even when their jobs aren't at stake—which, alas, they sometimes are—they act as if having diabetes is something to be ashamed of.

My doctor tells me that a good number of people well-known in the entertainment world are diabetic, but with the shining exception of Dan Rowan, they won't allow their names to used in conjunction with any diabetic fund-raising drives, because they feel it would damage their images. It is, in fact, much easier to learn about a movie star's sexual aberrations than it is to find out about the activity of his pancreas.

It was only after I began brazenly flaunting my own "guilty secret" that people confessed to me that they, too, bore the same stigma. Even at the beginning, though, everyone was quick to tell me encouraging tales about an aunt or a cousin or a neighbor who had had "it" and yet lived to be eighty-three or seventy-eight or ninety-two or some such triumphant geriatric pinnacle. Frankly, this well-meaning intelligence didn't thrill me. I wasn't so much worried about quantity as quality; I didn't feel as concerned with how long I was going to live as with how well I was going to live. If I was going to have to give up gourmet dining and wining and travel and sports and everything else that was a part of the active life I enjoyed, it was going to be like that old joke, "You may not live to be a hundred; it will just *seem* that long."

Since I had no one to talk to about my problem, I did as a good librarian should. I went to books for help. But for the first time in my life, they let me down. To paraphrase Emily Dickinson, there were no frigates like the books on diabetes to make me feel all at sea—in fact, almost sunk.

In the first place, they all sounded as if they had been written about the year of the discovery of insulin, and incidentally the year of my birth, 1922. The illustrations were not just poor, they were grisly or ludicrous. One of my favorites showed three nurses in high-button shoes and black stockings, standing together on a beam scales, grinning and looking like chorus girls from an early musical version of the life of Florence Nightingale.

Even the books that were a bit more up-to-date had one unpleasant trait in common. They would cheerfully announce at the outset that "a diabetic can lead a perfectly normal life," and then the rest of the book would be spent outlining how abnormal a diabetic's life really is. For one thing, someone leading a normal life isn't continually fiddling with his urine, nor does he as a matter of course observe any of the following admonitions that I read in the diabetes books:

Measure your food.
Never overeat.
Do not eat between meals.
Do not drink alcoholic beverages.
Exercise the same amount every day and only immediately after a meal.
Avoid emotional stress.
Do not sit with legs crossed.
After a shower, dry your ear canals with a cotton applicator.
Do not get sunburned.
Care for hangnails at once.
Do not shave your legs with a steel razor.
Do not use iodine.

Have someone else cut your toenails.
Do not walk barefoot.
Always use a shoehorn when putting on your shoes.
Wash your feet twice daily.
Massage your feet daily with alcohol or lanolin.
Do not use a hot-water bottle or heating pad or any heating
device on your feet.

A normal life, my foot! But what was I going to do? Although
I didn't want to go blind or drop dead of myocardial infarctions
or succumb to any other of the delights that are held out as
the wages of diabetic sinning, neither did I want to live like a
Tibetan ascetic.

While I knew that I couldn't ignore diabetes and hope it
would go away, neither was I going to take it lying down,
figuratively or literally. I decided that for me there was no
choice but to do battle with diabetes. Fortunately, in my campaign I had an enthusiastic and able aide-de-camp in Barbara.
She was, in fact, a more daring strategist than I—but then
she wasn't fighting on her own home ground. It wasn't the
castle of her skin that was under siege. But as it turned out,
the combination of her derring-do and my discretion struck an
effective balance.

Now that the smoke has cleared away from my two-year
campaign, I am happy to state that every battle but one has
been a victory, in fact, a near rout for our side. The one defeat,
although at the time I considered it my Waterloo, turned out to
be only a tactical retreat that gave me much needed reinforce-
ments for all future skirmishes.

Chapter 2

VALLEY
OF THE DOLLS

When I said before that all I knew about diabetes was that it had something to do with not eating sugar, that was not quite true. I did know one other thing, something I considered too obscene to think, much less talk, about. Diabetics have to stick needles into themselves. Regularly. Every bloody day.

The only pleasant event, therefore, of my St. Patrick's Day Diabetic Festival was the ceremony of the presentation of the Orinase pills and the information I gleaned from the accompanying book that the great majority of maturity-onset diabetics can get by either on diet alone or on a combination of diet and pills. Odious though having diabetes looked to be, I felt I could stand it as long as I didn't have to jab my flesh with the likes of what, judging by the illustrations in the diabetes books, could easily double at the race track for doping purposes. The descriptions of caring for syringes and needles and all the rest of the injection paraphernalia, along with the insulin itself, sounded as complicated and time-consuming as caring for a newborn infant:

> Sterilize syringes and needles by boiling them for five minutes.
> Check tip of syringe for chips.
> Check needle for burrs.
> Boil syringe in vinegar water when it becomes coated with lime.
> Clean the bore of the needle with wire.

No, I simply couldn't face the prospect of fitting all those needle nursemaid duties into my already glove-tight schedule.

But I wasn't terribly worried. After all, the odds were very much in my favor.

And so it was with a good full measure of confidence that I started in on my Orinase and urine-testing program. The first ten days (March 17–27) the doctor had me on two Orinase a day, one before breakfast and one before dinner. I was instructed to test my urine two hours after each meal. Sugar to some extent, and usually to some great extent, invariably appeared. My first days on Orinase were a thumping failure. But still I wasn't disturbed. The doctor had explained that he was starting me out slowly. I still had a long way to go before the single hair which suspended the diabetic needle of Damocles over my head would be cut.

I called in on March 27 to report. The doctor, seemingly unconcerned about my initial failure on oral compounds, upped the pills to two before breakfast and two before dinner. My record did not improve. So I gave the doctor's office another call on March 29. The doctor himself was not available, but the nurse called back and relayed the message that I was to raise the dosage to two Orinase before breakfast, two before lunch, and one before dinner. She then delivered an exit line pure Grand Guignol in horror: "If that doesn't work, the doctor says to come down on Friday and we'll show you how to use the needle."

Had I not been at the library reference desk at the time, I would have let forth a piercing scream. As it was, I ran, not walked, to the periodicals room to try to diminish the shock by sharing it with Barbara. In the sepulchral voice I use for delivering bad news (Barbara calls it my "tone *funeste*"), I announced to her, "I may have to take a fix." This was the merry term we used for going onto the needle in those halcyon days when I thought there was little chance that I'd ever have to.

Barbara looked as stricken as if she had just lost her best friend, which was gratifying, but hardly reassuring. Clutching my arm with a hand as clammy as my own, she pulled me back to the staff lounge and began the first of what has become a relentless series of interminable lectures, which she delivers *ex cathedra*, as if she were the holder of the Diabetic Chair at the Johns Hopkins School of Medicine.

"Doctors *can* be wrong, you know," she said, citing her own near brush with the scalpel when one doctor insisted on an exploratory operation on a cherished portion of her anatomy, while the second she consulted—an experienced surgeon in the field—dismissed the lump as a cyst and sent her about her business unsliced.

"You must," she ranted on, "get another medical opinion, an expert on diabetes. Tom will find you one. He knows all the best medical men." Tom is her husband and, as a lawyer who specializes in workmen's compensation, every day he deals with doctors as expert witnesses. Consequently, he's garnered a collection of pretty sharp Arrowsmiths.

In my already psychologically weakened state, I was in no condition to argue. I agreed to let Tom select a doctor and make an appointment for me. Of course, there *was* still the chance that the increased Orinase dosage would take hold in the next three days.

It didn't. So I bade my health service a not too reluctant and yet not too hypocritical farewell. "I want to find a doctor with more time . . . one who can work with me a little more closely. Please thank Dr. X for all his help."

On the following Wednesday, when I had an afternoon appointment with Tom's recommendation, a remarkable kismety, ESP-ish thing happened. Barbara was flipping through some of the newly arrived magazines in the periodicals department of the library. For some reason, that day the fates directed her to the *AMA Journal*, a publication she says she never reads except to glance at the cover to see if her favorite column, "The Fracture of the Month," is included. The fates this time had her thumb through and pulled her eyeballs to a full-color ad for the latest oral compound for diabetes, Tolinase. She read it, and even through the protective coating of medicalese was able to figure out that Tolinase was often successful with maturity-onset diabetics who had flunked out on Orinase.

She showed the ad to me and I agreed to ask the doctor if Tolinase might possibly work. I was, I admit, just doing it to humor her. I really held out small hope. But to my jubilant surprise, I returned from the doctor's office with the verdict that

I could try it for a few weeks to see if it could bring me under control.

Tolinase was an immediate improvement. A single one of them (100 mg.) before breakfast could lighten the green of my Tes-Tape more often that five Orinase ever did. And when the dosage was increased to one and a half (150 mg.), I was at last a happy dweller in the realms of buttercup-yellow Tes-Tape.

The only unfortunate effect of the success of Tolinase was that it convinced Barbara she was a natural combination of Madame Curie, Dr. Janet Travell, and Dr. Frances Kelsey, and consequently an incontrovertible authority on every known and unknown aspect of diabetes. Insufferable though this was, I could accept it with good grace because of my relief and happiness at having brought my disease under control with an oral drug.

Over the next few months the more I read about diabetes the more grateful I was that I had been able to avoid "taking a fix." Aside from the elements of fear of pain and aesthetic repugnance to the needle and the nuisance of taking care of the equipment, a diabetic on insulin has to eat his meals on a highly rigid time schedule and he daily faces the very real danger of going into shock. Although pill-takers occasionally get slight hypoglycemic twinges, they don't usually get the fall-down-pass-out reaction of full-blown "fitting" (a term Barbara and I use in much the same spirit as "taking a fix"). So whenever I got depressed or discouraged with my diabetic lot, I always cheered myself up with the comforting thought, "Well, at least I have escaped the needle."

The story of how I made it on the pills is a great little happy-ending melodrama, isn't it? As Thelma Ritter said in *All About Eve*, it has everything except the bloodhounds biting at my rear end. But stay, the bloodhounds are there waiting in the wings and my rear end is soon to be in imminent danger.

My honeymoon with Tolinase lasted from April until December, but after nine months of having it yellow-taped, I began to feel uneasy stirrings:

Item: After spending a rather damp week in Hawaii, I picked
    up a cold and spilled sugar all the way home.

Item: During a week in the mountains I engaged in strenuous physical exercise and lost three more pounds from my already inadequately fleshed frame.

Item: I started coming up with more than occasional green tapes. They would mysteriously appear, then clear up, then appear again.

But the strangest item of all was the business of the ketones (poisonous acids). When I got a deep green Tes-Tape, I would follow the recommended procedure of testing for ketones, too, and sometimes I would find them. But since I am an inveterate urine tester, I would occasionally also test for ketones when the tape was *negative,* and once in a while I would find slight hints of them then, too. And finally, on a weekend trip to Laguna Beach, I picked up a twinge of diarrhea. My Tes-Tape remained yellow, but my ketone test was not just positive, it was *peremptory.*

I discussed this baffling circumstance with Barbara, and for once her medical instincts failed her. "It can't be," she said. "Ketones," she quoted knowledgeably, "are an indication that you're heading into acidosis and toward diabetic coma, but how can you be heading toward diabetic coma if you aren't spilling sugar in your urine?"

I shrugged. "All I know is I have ketones."

"I guess you'd better talk to your doctor."

"I guess I'd better."

By this date I had changed to my third doctor, one nearer my home, and it was almost time for me to take my twenty-four-hour urine specimen to his office and have my regular bimonthly examination; so I waited until then. After the doctor had checked me over and sent me into the lab for a blood sugar test, he told me that from the looks of my urine test and my Tes-Tape record, which was well within his safety zone of not spilling more than 30 percent of the time, he thought I was all right. He said he'd call me when he had the results of my blood sugar test.

When he did telephone, he told me my blood sugar was a little over 200. Not good. I'd better up my Tolinase dosage to

350 mg. a day and then come in for another blood sugar test. Quite a jump from 150 mg. a day, I thought. He certainly didn't believe in sneaking up on it the way the other doctor had.

I did as directed. Three days later the blood test I took still revealed too much sugar. The doctor put the Tolinase dosage up even higher. Still I had not much green on my Tes-Tape, but still I was manufacturing ketones. The doctor prescribed a combination of Tolinase and Diabinese, another of the oral hypoglycemic agents. High blood sugar. Diabinese alone. High blood sugar. Still another hypoglycemic, DBI-TD. And one more blood sugar test.

All through this I was confident I would get by on some oral drug or other. (There are, after all, five varieties of them.) After chugging along on pills for almost a year, I couldn't believe they would let me down now. I reasoned that it was merely a question of finding the right combination or of getting rid of the vestiges of whatever intestinal infection it was that had stirred things up in the first place.

When the ax fell, it was fast but not painless. Again I was on duty in the library and it was late on a Friday afternoon, when the doctor called. "I'm still not satisfied with your blood sugar," he said, "and I think the only way we can handle it is with a little insulin. Can you come in after work and let the lab assistant show you how to give an injection?"

"This afternoon?" I begged off. I couldn't face it. My excuse was that Barbara and I were giving a talk for a writers' club that night in Manhattan Beach and there simply would not be time enough for me to stop by and learn how to use the needle and get to the lecture on time.

"All right. Can you come tomorrow morning? Early tomorrow morning?"

"Yes. I guess I can."

Barbara was not in the library. She was, in fact, several miles away, in Hollywood in a soundproof booth reading for Recording for the Blind. Totally inaccessible. There was nothing for me to do but go home alone and sit and stare and let the waves of woe wash over me.

When she got back and called to casually inquire if I'd heard anything from the doctor, I told her—and my tone had never been so *funeste*—that we couldn't go to Hawaii anymore.

"What?"

"I said Hawaii is out. I won't be able to wear a bathing suit from now on."

"What *are* you talking about?"

"My legs will be too scarred. I . . . I . . . have to go on the needle tomorrow."

Barbara dropped the phone and Mustanged over to my apartment, scoring the first half-minute mile in the Sherman Oaks record book.

Our preparations for delivering our hilarious speech on humor writing that night consisted of a couple of hours of weeping and wailing and tearing our hair like members of a Greek chorus. How we survived the talk neither of us remembers, but we're certain we must have caused any incipient humor writers in the audience to abandon the idea forever, scared off by the way it seemed to have turned us into the most dismal and morose of living creatures.

The next morning, under a typical Southern California overcast harbinger-of-smog sky, we went into the Saturday-deserted medical center building. The lab technician, Rae, whom I already knew very well from the recent weeks of bloodletting, gave me the doctor's prescription for U-40 NPH insulin and a box of disposable needles and syringes. We picked these up in the building's drugstore.

Back in the office I explained to Rae that I wanted Barbara to come in with me so she could learn the technique, too. She had volunteered to inject me when we were on trips or when I wore out all the sticking spots I could reach.

In the small bottle- and tube-lined lab, I was seated on a metal stool and instructed to make my left thigh available. Rae unwrapped the needle and syringe. I was surprised at how really delicate it was. Not only was it far too small for horse-doping, but it looked inadequate even for hyping up a sluggish greyhound.

"Who wants to do it?" Rae asked cheerily. She looked from one of us to the other while we each shrank beneath her eyes.

Rae sighed and said, "All right, I'll do it this time."

Lecturing all the while on what she was doing, she peeled the seal off the insulin bottle, cleaned the top with a piece of alcohol-soaked cotton, removed the plastic cover from the needle, exercised the plunger a bit to loosen it, pulled it back to slightly beyond the fifteen-unit mark to fill it with air, and stabbed it into the rubber top of the insulin bottle. She then pushed the plunger in all the way with her thumb and, bracing the syringe with her first two fingers, slowly sucked in fifteen units. "Be sure you don't have any air bubbles or you won't be getting the right amount of insulin." Out came the needle from the bottle.

"Now you pinch up the flesh and sterilize the spot. Then it's just like throwing a dart. See?"

Zap! The needle sank into my thigh. Although I winced and recoiled, I didn't feel a thing.

She left the needle just sticking in there—I guess so I could get used to the sight of it—while she chatted amiably about other possible injection spots. "The front and sides of the thigh, the upper arms, the lower part of the abdomen, the stomach, and the buttocks. Almost anywhere, really."

Taking hold of the syringe again, she continued with the demonstration. "First, you pull the plunger back a little, like this, to make sure you haven't hit a blood vessel. If you have, you'll see some blood come into the syringe. It almost never happens, though. The needles are too short to get down that far. Still, it's a good idea to check. It's the proper injection technique and you ought to be in the habit of doing it correctly in case you ever have to give anybody some other kind of shot. Anyway, if you should get blood, just pull it out and start over."

"What happens if you forget to check and it turns out you're in a blood vessel?" Barbara asked.

"Oh, nothing too bad. It just means the insulin goes directly into the bloodstream and hits you faster than usual.

"OK," she went on with the lesson. "Now you push the plunger in all the way. Take out the needle and press the injection spot with your alcohol-soaked cotton and that's it."

Barbara and I released our mutually held breath. There was my thigh—perfect for exposure on the sands of Waikiki.

"Do you think you can do it now?" Rae asked.

"I guess I don't have any choice," I said.

Barbara, whose eyes looked unnaturally bright and whose tongue was unnaturally still, nodded a weak affirmative.

On the way home we stopped in at the market and picked up a couple of thick-skinned navel oranges. Back at my apartment, before we settled down for one of the least productive of our writing sessions, we spent about an hour reviewing the technique and jabbing the bright round orange abdomens.

When Barbara was leaving at the end of the day she drew herself up and, fixing a noble Sidney Carton "It is a far, far better thing I do than I have ever done" expression on her face, said, "I'll come over in the morning and give you your first fix."

Tempted though I was, I was firm. "No, I have to learn to do it myself and tomorrow's the time to start."

That night it was a far, far worse rest I went to than I had ever known.

I got up unusually early. There was no point in just lying there writhing. I got all the equipment. Then I tried to remember everything Rae had said. I had to go almost exclusively by her instructions because, despite my vast reading on the subject of diabetes, I had always skipped the paragraphs—and especially the pictures—about injections. All I really knew was what I had learned from the demonstration.

Not feeling up to breaking totally fresh injection-site ground, I aimed for about the same spot Rae had, except on the other thigh, and with the strength and determination of Brutus doing in Caesar, I gritted my teeth, narrowed my eyes, and stabbed. It slipped in like a fork into mashed potatoes. An orange, I found, is much tougher than a human. The only thing I felt was the front end of the syringe touching my skin. The needle might as well not even have been there.

I pushed the plunger, pressed the spot with the alcohol-soaked cotton as I removed the needle, and *voilà*, all done. Triumph! Exultation! Cockiness!

The next day, when I reported to the doctor, he asked me how I was doing with the needle. Preening shamelessly, I announced, "Superbly. Nothing to it."

But if I felt an overweening pride at my accomplishment, I was a candidate for the modesty trophy compared to Barbara, when she gave me my shot for the first time. I've never seen anyone approach a project with greater trepidation or emerge with greater jubilation. From then on she referred to herself as "Nurse Jane Fuzzy-Wuzzy, the kindly rabbit nurse," a favorite Uncle Wiggly character. Now whenever we travel together, she insists on giving the injection every day. "The Old Fuzz," she says with a firmness that leaves no room for argument, "will give you your fix."

But, diabetic, what of the curative power of insulin? How did it work? Beautifully! During that first week of what seemed to be wanton dining, I gained back seven of my lost pounds. The doctor and I decided that what I had been doing during the last few months on the pills was starving myself. That's why there had been ketones without sugar in the urine. Although it seemed I had been eating an adequate amount of *food*, I had subconsciously been cutting down on my carbohydrates, the way a follower of the so-called "drinking man's diet" would do. Only I carried it to an extreme. In managing not to have carbohydrates to spill on, I wound up not having enough to run a body on. My system was literally devouring itself. In retrospect, I'm only amazed that I didn't manage to get even worse reactions from this little fasting excursion. I've read, for example, that those people who go on the sleep diet, where they knock you out for a few days, often develop the gout from consuming their own flesh.

On insulin my energy picked up tremendously and my appearance improved to the point that people began to say, "You're looking wonderful," and *mean* it. In my skeletal days, friends would stare at me in disbelief at the change that diabetes had wrought and, feeling compelled to say something, would usually gush out a compliment that was as overdone as it was insincere.

My only regret now is that I didn't go on insulin sooner. My doctor tells me that many other patients say the same thing. I wouldn't have been satisfied, though, if I hadn't first given the pills every chance to bring my blood sugar down, because being on insulin *is* a bit more inconvenient. But only a bit. I've never yet boiled a syringe or cleaned the bore of a needle with a wire or rinsed anything in alcohol or checked anything for chips or burrs, and I never intend to. To my mind, the individually packaged disposable needles and syringes rank along with deodorant for men as one of the greatest inventions of the twentieth century. Becton, Dickinson and Johnson and Johnson both make them. They cost less than half a pack of cigarattes a day, including the insulin, which is often less than what the pill-takers have to put out for their daily treatment. Disposable needles and syringes have the additional advantage of letting you know if you've taken your injection or not. For people who tend to be absentminded or for those so used to injecting themselves with insulin that it's done automatically, it's a comfort, when it suddenly occurs to you, "Did I or didn't I?" to be able to look in the wastebasket for visible evidence one way or the other.

I won't pretend that taking a fix is always a joy pop for me, though. On some groggy mornings I fumble and botch. I'm especially poor at jabbing in the soft underbelly, tending to instinctively pull back at the last minute. It's like anything else—you can, after all, even do a poor job of brushing your teeth and wind up with a sore gum.

Still, being on the needle is most definitely not misery. Misery is needing to go on the needle and not doing it. For, while my official diabetic classification is now insulin-dependent, I prefer to think of myself as insulin-*independent*. It is insulin that makes it possible for me to go on living exactly the kind of life I choose.

Chapter 3

THERE'S A
DOCTOR IN YOUR HOUSE

Most people feel they're married to their doctors. For them it is, to use a macabre metaphor, a 'til-death-do-us-part relationship. It must seem, therefore, that I am indeed a fickle sort, since I have been practicing a medical version of what they call these days "serial polygamy." In other words, in my short diabetic life I've had three different doctors. I divorced two of them with no regrets, and I think that we all remain good friends and bear each other no ill will.

I've explained why I left Dr. No. 1. With Dr. No. 2 the parting was more difficult. The first time I saw him, when I came in with my idea of trying Tolinase, he didn't laugh in my face, nor did he high-handedly ask where I went to medical school that I should be prescribing my own medication. No, he just said we'd try it, because with diabetes you never know what's going to work. This immediately gave me confidence in him. It showed that he had enough confidence in himself not to have to play the role of infallible medical oracle to impress me.

The Tolinase worked and I found happiness with Dr. No. 2. But soon small storm clouds began to form on our horizon. Tom was right. Dr. No. 2 was an excellent physician. In fact, he was so excellent that he was apparently used by *all* the workmen's compensation attorneys. It was difficult to contact him by telephone; and it was difficult to get a fast appointment with him. Also, his office was located over the hills and far away from the San Fernando Valley. A medical appointment with him could take as long as three hours portal to portal. This driving distance, combined with his busy schedule, gave me feelings of disquietude. What would I do if I ever had one of those des-

21

perate emergencies books on diabetes are always describing in ghastly detail?

The third ground, the one that eventually led to my divorce from him, was that, although he was a cardiovascular man and that is closely related to diabetes, it still didn't seem to me to be right on target. Diabetes was not really his medical bag, his own thing, and he couldn't possibly find it as delectably fascinating as I did.

As I am in the habit of doing, however, I merely stewed and complained about all this to Barbara, but I made no move. And as she is in the habit of doing, she lost patience with me and decided to take over herself. She called what were rapidly becoming her old friends at the local diabetes association and asked if they had a list of doctors in the Los Angeles area who specialized in diabetes. They did. Were there any in the San Fernando Valley? There were. Three of them. Could she have the names and addresses? Of course. And kismet strikes again: One of these three was located in a medical building only four blocks from where I live and right on the route I take daily to the college.

Since propinquity is usually as good a reason as any for starting up a relationship, I consented to make an appointment to see if this doctor and I would turn out to be compatible. Here I would like to mention that divorcing a doctor, like divorcing a husband, is an expensive proposition in both time and money. This is because the new doctor insists—and this is quite understandable—on giving a complete physical examination and taking down a total medical history. Consequently, during my initial diabetic year of doctor-changing I was as thoroughly and frequently examined as an astronaut, but unfortunately the government was not picking up the bills.

Right off in my initial appointment with Dr. No. 3 I knew he was for me. He had a pleasant, unhurried manner and I could tell as he inquired into the details of my health that his thoughts were more like "Oh, boy, another fascinating case of diabetes," rather than the "Ho, hum, another boring diabetic" that I always feared went through doctors' minds.

My subtle inquiries to Dr. No. 3 revealed that he lectured on the subject of diabetes at the University of Southern California School of Medicine. Furthermore, he was a past president of the Diabetes Association of Southern California, and he had been instrumental in pushing through the rule change that made it possible for diabetics to be hired by my own employer, the Los Angeles City Schools. This had, incidentally, taken place only seven years earlier, an indication of how archaic attitudes about diabetics are still breathing hot on our necks.

What made Dr. No. 3 even more too-good-to-be-true was that I would in effect be getting two diabetes experts for the price of one. His associate was the immediate past president of the Diabetes Association of Southern California, and either one or the other of them was on twenty-four-hour call for any diabetic emergency that might arise. What a comfort this was, especially during the tense days later of flunking out on the pills and going onto insulin. Also, since Dr. No. 3 was an internist, he could look after my general welfare as he kept track of my specific malady.

One thing I've learned about specialists that surprised me is that rather than being extremely rigid in their treatment, they are more relaxed. For example, the doctor who had me toeing the mark the most in my diabetic regime was Dr. No. 1, an internist. Dr. No. 2, an internist with a cardiovascular specialty, which narrowed it down a little closer to diabetes, allowed me more latitude in diet and behavior. Dr. No. 3, the internist-diabetes specialist, is the least restrictive of all. I remember his answering one of my furrow-browed queries about diet and exercise regulation with, "Of course it would be ideal if you ate exactly the same amount every day of your life, and exercised exactly the same amount, and got exactly the same amount of sleep, but it would be impossible to control things that closely, even if you were a laboratory animal. And you're not, you're a human being and you have to live like one." These sentiments were echoed by another diabetes expert, Dr. Alvin L. Schultz, Professor of Medicine at the University of Minnesota, who, writing in *The Diabetic,* said, "Ideally, if all three factors, diet, exercise, and insulin, were constant from day to day, diabetic control should be perfect. Few diabetics find it possible, or even desirable, to lead such an orderly, rigid, and compulsive existence."

Although I would never advise anyone to change doctors if he felt well and looked well and *was* well, I did suggest to a diabetic friend of mine at the college whose diabetes was discovered about six months after mine that he go see Dr. No. 3, with whom I was so delighted. My diabetic friend was extremely unhappy on a regime that seemed quite laboratory-animalesque to me, and he looked more skeletal than I had in my darkest self-consuming days. He was, however, morally indignant at the mere thought of consulting another physician. "I can't change doctors," he explained. "Our family has gone to this man for years." In a case like this, it would seem to me that he could hold onto his old wife/doctor for sentimentality's sake and keep a mistress/diabetes specialist on the other side for happiness's sake. I don't even think his doctor would be offended, because, as I understand it, it's legitimate procedure for patients, as well as for doctors, to consult with more than one medical authority.

But what actually is good treatment? When I attended the diabetes fair in Los Angeles, I kept hearing questions from the audience that indicated that diabetics didn't know what to expect from their doctors. They had no idea whether they were getting poor, average, or excellent attention. Therefore, I'll outline here what my doctor does for me, since I consider myself to be under the very best of care.

First and foremost, Dr. No. 3 requires that I have an appointment with him every other month—as the Saturday-night-bath joke goes—whether I need one or not. At these appointments I am to bring in a twenty-four-hour urine specimen, and I am always given a blood sugar test, because blood sugar is the only positive indicator of how well your diabetes is controlled, as I learned the hard way.

The nurse starts off by weighing me. The doctor then checks my eyes. After that he and I have a talk about my general health. "How are you feeling? Any problems?" he asks, leaving himself wide open for any litany of complaints I may have put together over the previous two months. What I like most about Dr. No. 3 is that although his reputation is outstanding (other doctors

I've talked to always remark on his abilities) and I know he has a tight schedule, he never gives me the impression that he's in a hurry to hustle me out of the office and get to the next patient. I always feel I could sit there forever asking an endless string of questions.

He usually inquires how much sugar I've been spilling and checks over my urine and ketone records if I've brought them in. I only keep a written account these days if the pattern is puzzling.

During these interviews I frequently used to have him write out extra prescriptions for syringes and insulin, because I was operating on the false idea that many diabetics (and some doctors and pharmacists) have, that syringes and insulin require a prescription. Legally in California, where I live, they do not, but actually they often do. For example, two different pharmacists I've approached have not only required prescriptions but insisted on keeping them. Consequently, although I now don't offer prescriptions for these items to pharmacists, I still always carry a prescription for both in my wallet just to be on the safe side—always the best place for a diabetic to be.

I get the results of my blood sugar test the following day by telephone. Although it might not make any difference to some diabetics, what I particularly like is that the doctor quotes me the exact figure instead of mysteriously suppressing it and dismissing me with a "You're OK" or "Your blood sugar is fine." I am told that it is 100 or 125 or 200 or whatever, and I can compare my score with what I know to be the normal blood sugar range: 80–110. Should my blood sugar be higher or lower than normal, the doctor discusses the regulation of my insulin dosage with me. He signs off with "See you again in two months" just to imprint on my mind that I am to let him keep me under regular surveillance.

In the interim I have the twenty-four-hour emergency service at my disposal. Once around the Christmas holidays I started developing a sore throat. I dialed the number and within the hour my doctor's associate got in touch with me. I'd better add that I made it clear on the telephone that this was not a screaming emergency. Once when it was, the answering service held me on the line until they could put the doctor himself on, a matter of a three-minute interval. The doctor discussed my problem with me, called in a prescription to the nearest pharmacy, and I slew the germs before they got a toehold in my respiratory tract.

But ask not what your doctor can do for you; ask what you can do for your doctor. He has no way of interpreting your testing records unless you keep them and keep them regularly and accurately. He cannot answer your questions unless you ask them. Doctors, no matter how experienced and excellent, are not mind readers. Make notes, if you need to, but arrive at your appointment with a clear idea of what you want to tell your doctor and what you want to ask him. Even if he is the sort who gives you the impression that he has a limitless amount of time for you, he is an extremely busy man, and if you have any consideration at all, you won't make him sit there while you grope around in the shadowy corners of your mind trying to dredge up the questions you dropped there some time during the previous month or so.

Another way to help your doctor help you is to play it straight. Don't fake your records to disguise your sweet sessions of silent sugar sinning, if you have them. Don't eat casually for two months and then, on the day you know your blood sugar is being taken, adhere to your diet as closely as if you were a test case at a diabetes education and detection center. Maybe you think these cautions are unnecessary—and maybe for you they are—but I have it on good authority that we diabetics are known in the medical profession as the mad Hungarians. I know, because an orthopedist I consulted once for a knee problem probed deeply into my diabetic regime and then summed up his impressions with: "You're the first sensible diabetic I've ever met."

In diabetes more than in any other disease the doctor can only help those who help themselves. There is a very distinct limit to what the doctor can do for you. The basic diabetic treatment is done by you yourself and done daily. Diabetes is the great do-it-yourself disease. And doing it yourself takes discipline and education, much of it self-education. Your doctor cannot pop around every day and hand you your pills or give you your injection. Your doctor cannot plan your meals and see that you eat them. Your doctor cannot lead you off to the golf course or the bowling alley or take you for a walk so you'll get the proper exercise. Your doctor cannot tuck you into bed each night and watch over you to see that you get your eight hours' sleep. And he certainly can't dwell within your skin and note the unusual reactions and feelings that indicate something may be amiss. No, even if you had Banting and Best and Joslin living with you and standing eight-hour shifts, you would still have to rely on yourself to take care of yourself, because in diabetes you are the doctor. Physician, heal thyself.

Chapter 4

I AM A DIABETIC;
I AM NOT INTOXICATED

Knock three times and ask for Joe before continuing. This is a bootleg chapter. It probably could not win the ADA seal of approval, unless you use ADA to stand for the American Distillers' Association rather than American Diabetes Association. For drinking, according to the editor of the *ADA Forecast*, is still "medically controversial." I'm tempted to reply, "When it comes to diabetes, what isn't?" At any rate, I come neither to bury drinking nor to praise it, but merely to tell what *I* did and do, with no go-thou-and-do-likewise implications.

When people ask me what I did when my doctor told me I wasn't to do any drinking with diabetes, I like to respond, "I changed doctors." This is, of course, a facetious answer with only a few units of truth in it.

It is true, however, that my first doctor did forbid drinking. In fact, one of my most vivid remembrances of the day on which he revealed to me that I had diabetes for sure is of being handed the 1,800-calorie exchange list, glancing through the general rules, and spotting under "Foods to Avoid" the words "beer, wine, or other alcoholic beverages." I recall giving a dry gulp and saying squeakily to the doctor, "No alcohol at all?"

He peered at me over his glasses as if inspecting me for scarlet veins on my nose or other signs of incipient dipsomania and asked, rather unsympathetically, I thought, "Is that going to be so hard on you?"

"No," I said, not entirely honestly, "but it's going to be pretty hard on my friends."

That night as I had dinner with Barbara and Tom, I drank my "last martini" and my "last glass of wine" along with my

28

"last" uncalculated servings of carbohydrous foods. I intended to start my diet the next day, but I might just as well have begun my new regime that night for all the pleasure I got out of the dining and drinking experience. Everything I swallowed had trouble working its way past the large lump that had formed about halfway down my esophagus. Having negotiated that hazard, my food plopped with almost an echo into my fear-hollowed stomach. Barbara and Tom, too, seemed caught up in the last-supper mood as they alternated between a false it's-not-so-bad, look-on-the-bright-side gaiety and tight-lipped silence.

The next day I began my temperance regime—temperance in the sense that most temperance workers define it: total abstinence. I immediately understood why people who can take it or leave it alone seldom elect to leave it alone. I missed the cocktail before dinner not so much for the alcohol itself as for the relaxed atmosphere it seems to create, that unwinding effect.

I missed the glass of wine with dinner, again not so much for its alcohol content as for its synergistic combination with the food, its ability to turn a creature necessity into one of the delights of civilization.

But my original remark to my doctor had been correct. If it bothered me, it bothered my friends even more. Especially Barbara. Some of our best thinking had been done during cocktail hours and leisurely wine-lubricated meals. Here I want to emphasize *thinking*, not writing. Neither of us can compose a decent sentence after so much as a teaspoonful of cough syrup. But at the end of the day, when the actual writing is finished and new ideas and angles are being groped for, a drink and the atmosphere it creates serve to unleash the mind and let it wander freely in meadows where it might stumble upon something original.

The tranquilizing effect of the alcohol was another lack we felt. In the words of a sympathetic literary agent we know, "As a tension-producing activity, writing is second only to scuba diving." And although our writing is usually more of the light variety, the kind that, if successful, sounds as if we "just sat down and dashed it off" (as one of our less tactful acquaintances once put it), we anguish over our semicolons along with the best of them, and at the end of the day the bolts in the back of our necks are as tight as any.

Abruptly, all our lovely end-of-the-workday mind-in-the-meadows tranquillity came to an end. There was no cocktail hour interlude, and the dinner-table conversation was limited to grouchy comments by Barbara that I had eaten only a *third* of a cup of squash instead of the half-cup that the exchange list dictated, or that I was supposed to eat five more grapes—as she covered the paper on the clipboard, not with book and article ideas as formerly, but with computations of calories, carbohydrates, fats, and proteins.

Although I urged her to, Barbara refused to continue having her cocktail while I had Diet-Rite or some such noncarbohydrous, nonalcoholic liquid, saying that it would be "a travesty" and protesting that "it's no fun to drink alone" and "it wouldn't work." Indeed, I knew it wouldn't. One mind can hardly loosen up and skip about while the other one is sitting stolidly with its arms folded, blocking the way with thoughts only of the mathematics of the meal ahead.

The sole drink I had during this drought was on one of the nights of our diabetes-shakedown trip to Yosemite, when I pretended that Barbara had convinced me that just one drink wouldn't hurt anything. As I silently and nervously sipped at a bourbon and water, I imagined I could feel the blood vessels popping in my eyeballs and hear the anguished screams of my abused pancreas. As a result, our cocktail hour had all the hilarity of a hemlock-tasting party.

Even though this initial timid diabetic handshake with John Barleycorn could hardly have been called a *succès fou*, at least it didn't make me drop to the floor in a coma, as I expected it might. In fact, as far as I could tell, except for its ravaging of my conscience, it didn't affect me adversely in any way at all.

It also encouraged Barbara to step up her soft-sell one-drink-before-dinner campaign. She began inserting her "So-and-so drinks and so-and-so is a diabetic" sentence into the conversation even more frequently than before. "Jim Barrett drinks and *he's* a diabetic," she'd say, citing one of her husband's friends whose diabetes was activated in the Air Force. (A dandy place to get it, incidentally, since, although he looks as fit as a Stradivarius, his particular case involved a 40 'percent disability pension—enough to keep him in platinum needles and Baccarat syringes the rest of his life.)

She also started leaving open on the coffee table Bill Talbert's *Playing for Life*, with passages underlined such as: "What was wrong with my wanting one more drink in one more bar? A few scotches in an evening—did that make me a drunk? Had I ever shown the slightest sign that I couldn't handle it?"

I remained rigid, though. Whenever Barbara trotted out her ubiquitous "So-and-so drinks and so-and-so is a diabetic," I would always snappily rejoin, "Yes, and Brendan Behan drank and he *was* a diabetic." I didn't really back this up with much conviction, though, because I knew there was more than a slight difference between my proposed one cocktail and Behan's roaring boy-o regular twenty-four-hour pub-a-thons.

And the more we read on the subject of diabetes, the more I, too, became convinced that, indeed, one little drink wouldn't do me any harm. For example, in *How to Live with Diabetes* (by Henry Dolger, M.D., and Bernard Seeman) we found the cheerful tidings that "this does not mean that the average adult diabetic must abstain from alcohol for medical reasons. On the contrary, circumstances exist where alcohol is useful in diabetes." And in the Ames Company publication *Diabetes in the News* there was an item headed "It Is a Fact: Good News for Persons with Diabetes," which read:

> Dr. Chauncey D. Leake and Dr. Milton Silverman in their new book, *Alcoholic Beverages in Clinical Medicine,* just published for physicians, state "dry table wines, which are low in sugar, have been found particularly useful in diabetes and have been widely prescribed, both to provide a readily utilizable source of food energy . . . and to brighten what may be a restricted diet. . . ."

For those who are interested in historical sidelights, we were, surprised to discover in our research that alcohol was one of the mainstays of the diabetic diet originated in the last century by the great specialist Apollinaire Bouchardat. Since alcohol is converted into energy without insulin, he used it to replace carbohydrates in the diet of diabetics. Ah, those French!

The British, too, have a far more relaxed attitude than we about drinking for diabetics. Not only does the British Diabetic Association publish under its imprimatur a leaflet giving the carbohydrate count of several alcoholic beverages—including seven (7!) kinds of ale and beer—but also, in their foreign travel brochure under the subject of wines, they say:

> It certainly seems a great pity to be on the Continent and not to enjoy this cheap and pleasant accompaniment to a meal. Unless you are overweight a glass of wine is a practical proposition, since it is very easy to get a dry wine in which the carbohydrate is negligible.

Not that there aren't problems involved with a diabetic's drinking, but they are mostly peripheral. For instance, some people might lack self-control after a drink, have another, postpone dinner, wander off toward home alone, topple over in insulin shock and, since they would have alcohol on their breath, perhaps wind up in the drunk tank to sleep off something unsleep-offable. This would be highly unlikely as far as I was concerned because I would definitely have no more than one drink—as Barbara hyperbolically puts it, "June's self-control is such that by comparison Gandhi would appear a wanton"— and also I only proposed to drink at home within reaching distance of the dinner table or, if out, in the company of someone who knew my situation.

Then, too, there is the problem that alcohol gives calories without food value. This could cause complications in overweight and poor nutrition cases. Again this wouldn't apply to me. Not only was my diet perfectly balanced—I was almost a fanatic on that—but I had always been as thin as a venetian-blind slat, and my diabetic regime had caused me to drop another two dress sizes, making me look positively cadaverous. I needed extra calories, especially calories without carbohydrates, any way I could get them.

While all this ratiocination mixed with rationalization was going on, I had changed doctors. Not because I was trying to find one who'd approve of drinking, as my little joke has it, but because of the needle-avoidance and specialist-seeking I've already explained. I had never asked this new doctor about drinking, probably because subconsciously I was afraid he'd say no.

Finally Barbara insisted. "Look, just ask him *why* you can't have one crummy drink before dinner. Since you're so underweight, the calories couldn't do any harm, and we know you're not going to skip dinner and pass out. If he can give you one logical reason why you shouldn't, if it might seriously affect your health in any way, I'll stop nagging. I swear it. In fact I won't *let* you take a drink when I'm around."

So, structuring the query with quotes and pointings out of the obvious, that is, my growing gauntness, I posed The Question to my doctor. He frowned and reluctantly admitted that as far as it went my reasoning was correct. There was, however, an additional consideration. The alcohol might upset the balance with the medication. "You would," the doctor explained, "have to drink regularly about the same amount each day to keep on an even keel." (Not that the doctor *advised* drinking in this manner, mind you.) I was jubilant. A small amount each day was all I ever wanted.

Now that I had what, by making use of a highly elasticized imagination, I could call "my doctor's approval," Barbara and I began to investigate just what varieties of alcohol and cocktail concoctions would be permissible. Since I was still on the pills at the time and, consequently, was still shucking off weight, calories posed no problem, but naturally carbohydrates did. Information on certain drinks was not at all hard to find: bourbon, scotch, rye, rum, gin, vodka, and cognac all had no carbohydrates. Others we could find nowhere: dinner wines, dessert wines, fruit-flavored brandies, brand-name liqueurs. And still others were given widely conflicting reports. Beer, for instance, was assigned two grams of carbohydrate per eight-ounce glass in Helen and Joseph Rosenthal's *Diabetic Care in Pictures* (3rd ed., Lippincott, 1960, p. 219) while in Bowes and Church's *Food Values of Portions Commonly Used* (10th ed., Lippincott, 1966, p. 7) the same-size glass was given 10.6 carbohydrates. After researching all available guides and writing to various distillers, we have managed to compile our own list (see Appendix B), which is as complete and accurate as our combined library vocations and imbibing avocations can make it.

What and how much do I drink now? Generally before dinner I have one of those drinks which contain no carbohydrate—either a martini or bourbon on the rocks. For variety I sometimes have a pseudo–old-fashioned, which is an old-fashioned made without either sugar, the maraschino cherry, or the orange slice. Occasionally, Barbara stirs me up a daiquiri or a gimlet made with fresh lime juice and artificial sweetener. Whatever I have, I scrupulously measure one 1½-ounce jigger of the alcohol, or I observe mine host carefully to make sure he doesn't, out of a misguided sense of generosity, slosh in a little extra. (Yet another reason not to trust a man mixing drinks.) Fortunately, in bars I never have to worry about getting more than one strict measure!

When I dine with Barbara or when I have guests or when I am a guest, I also have a glass (about 3½ ounces) of dry wine with dinner. On state occasions after dinner I sometimes have a bit (about half as much as a regular portion) of cognac or, if I need extra carbohydrates, a liqueur such as Benedictine or Chartreuse.

In France I skip the hard liquor before dinner, preferring to have instead two or three glasses of wine with dinner, a white with the fish course and a red with the main course and the cheese course. Also, when in France I usually have a glass of wine with lunch, and my system seems to know where it is and to react accordingly. That is to say, it doesn't react at all.

On Saturdays and Sundays and holidays when I'm at home I often have a glass (half a can) of beer with lunch. And sometimes I put a tablespoon of rum for flavor into my before-bed milk.

Do I ever break my strict one-drink-before-dinner regime? Yes, but *very* occasionally and invariably for an important cause, such as having a conference with an editor when vital matters are being discussed and no one seems ready to order dinner. The two drinks I have in these circumstances are not only used to promote conviviality and concomitant contracts, but as survival kits as well. I always order Bloody Marys so the tomato can keep socking carbohydrates to me and I won't say or do anything foolish—or go goofy, as Barbara puts it—at a crucial moment. I also know that if I did, indeed, start going into insulin shock, I could easily substitute a screwdriver for a Bloody Mary and there would be the instant recovery that orange juice is famous for.

Again, let me assure you that this wanton two-drink binge occurs only a couple of times a year and only in New York (wicked city) and always with Nurse Jane Fuzzy-Wuzzy in attendance, her purse full of crackers and sugar cubes.

And now that I've ticked off my drinking habits, I realize that when written out and concentrated in a couple of paragraphs they sound a lot wilder than they are. It's as I once heard Ilka Chase say when discussing one of her travel books on TV. She confessed that when she was revising the manuscript, she had to cut out several of the references to "we stopped at a little cafe and had a glass of . . ." because it sounded as if they did nothing but reel from one drink to another.

My drinking pattern is small amounts taken regularly and drunk slowly. Since I've been diabetic, I've never had so much as an incipient numb upper lip—for me the sign of beginning to feel alcohol. More through personal preference than diabetic restriction, I never go to cocktail parties if I can avoid them, that is to say, unless they're for business or duty. I never go to wee-hours, big-bash parties under any circumstances, again out of personal preference. No Bill Talbert I. I still get a thrill of horror when I read his descriptions of all-night drinking and conga-dancing escapades:

> For the finals of the Land of Sky tennis tournament the next afternoon, I had to change directly from my dinner clothes into my white flannels. I had got back from the party only a couple of hours before, with just about time for a long cold shower in between.

There is an Oriental saying, "First the man takes a drink, then the drink takes a drink, then the drink takes the man," and if you're the kind of person whose first drink invariably takes a drink with the logical progression following, then I would say you would be utterly stupid as a diabetic to drink at all. In fact, you'd be utterly stupid as a nondiabetic to drink at all. I would further say that there are two very valid and sound reasons for a diabetic not to drink:

1. If drinking means nothing to you.
2. If drinking means everything to you.

And now, before we're raided, we'll close up this speakeasy, leaving it entirely up to you and your doctor whether or not you can in good conscience cast your vote for the repeal of prohibition.

Chapter 5

NOBODY KNOWS
THE TRUFFLES I'VE SEEN

A fair exchange is no robbery, but the exchange list diet **Dr. No.** 1 gave me along with my diabetic tidings struck me as a robbery of the magnitude of the Brink's heist. By limiting both what I could eat and how much I could eat, it stole away all dining pleasure, and by removing one of the best writing markets Barbara and I had—gourmet food and drink—it compounded the felony.

The gap between what I was used to eating and what was contained on the seven little food lists of the diet sheet was Grand Canyon-like. And yet there it was in boldface print: "Eat only those foods which are on diet list." *Only* those foods? *Only* those prosaic staples? No more lobster? No more guava juice? No more artichokes? No more water chestnuts? No more truffles? Obviously not, because not a single one of these had made the lists.

As Barbara said, "Why?"

"I guess, because the foods on the lists are the only ones that don't upset diabetics."

"Nonsense," she retorted from the depths of her diabetic ignorance, which was at that time exactly as profound as my own. "Look, shrimp's on the list, and what can lobster do to you that shrimp can't? Besides, what if you were Mexican? Couldn't you ever touch a tortilla again? Or if you were Jewish, would it be good-bye forever to matzo balls and bagels?"

"Don't ask me," I shrugged. "All I know is what I read on this paper."

But on thinking further, I realized that was not *quite* all I knew about the exchange lists. The doctor had made one comment, "You don't need to pay any attention to this," and he had

37

taken his pen and crossed out the boldface print that admonished, "Do not eat between meals."

This gave me a whiff of hope. If one restriction in boldface could be so easily wiped out, maybe others could, too. Maybe it was just that there wasn't enough space to put everything in, so the originators of the food exchange lists, the American Diabetes Association and the American Dietetic Association, had only included the most common foods. After all, there was another rule about "foods to avoid (sugar, candy, honey, jam, etc.)" and here were listed only about eighteen or so items. If these were the only foods you shouldn't eat and the seven exchange lists were the only foods you could eat, then what of the tremendous number of foods that fell in neither the you-can nor the you-can't group, what of that great gray limbo of foods that, diabetically, were neither fish nor fowl?

One of the best fringe benefits of working at a college is that you have a built-in staff of experts to consult. Taking advantage of this, I hied me over to the Home Economics Department, where to my extreme happiness and relief I found that the head of the department, Ida Jaqua, had formerly been a dietician at both Mt. Sinai Hospital and the City of Hope and consequently was a major expert on nutrition. She was quick to inform me that the areas which, according to the exchange list diet, were diabetic no-man's-land, were perfectly habitable to me. There was nothing inherently dangerous about any of the unmentioned foods. In fact, when you come right down to it, she told me, *all* foods are diabetic fodder. This truth I later found confirmed in "Diet and Diabetes," a pamphlet published by the British Diabetic Association:

> One of the commonest misunderstandings about the diabetic diet is the mistaken impression that a diabetic can never eat certain foods. Generally speaking, there is no food a diabetic cannot include in his diet PROVIDED THAT HE KNOWS AND TAKES INTO ACCOUNT ITS FOOD VALUE.

That's the clue. If you wander from the exchange lists, you have to know exactly what you're eating. Mrs. Jaqua put me onto two books of nutritional analysis that could tell me the value of almost every food I might want to eat: the U. S. Department of Agriculture's *Composition of Foods,* and *Food Values of Portions Commonly Used* by Bowes and Church (10th ed., Lippincott, 1960). This latter was a particular wonder. Although it didn't contain an analysis of truffles, it did have lobster and guava juice and artichokes and water chestnuts and tortillas and in addition such exotics as reindeer milk and raccoon meat (both raw and cooked). Who could ask for anything more?

Barbara and I leaped to the conclusion that we were home safe and sound around the dinner table. It's true that with these analyses I could eat at least limited quantities of virtually anything I wanted and still stick to my doctor's orders—1,800 calories a day, divided thus: 180 grams of carbohydrate, 80 grams of protein, and 80 grams of fat. But here was the hitch: in order to get the proper balance of calories, carbohydrates, proteins, and fats, we had to work out as many complex calculations as it would take to figure a moon shot.

I'll never forget how during that first week, when Barbara and I were dining in baronial splendor in the candle-lit great hall dining room of the Ahwahnee Hotel in Yosemite, I had to sit with Bowes and Church on my lap calling out numbers to her, while she tried to compute me a dinner on the spot from the menu the head waiter handed us.

Here's a sample of what just one meal's computations looked like:

DINNER	Calories	Protein	Fat	Carbohydrate
Lettuce salad	15	1.0g.	0.3g.	2.7g.
Salad dressing	10		5.0	
½ cup beets	34	0.8	0.1	8.1
½ cup spinach	23	2.8	0.6	3.3
2 teaspoons butter	72		8.2	
2 lamb chops	205	24.9	10.9	
1 slice bread	63	2.0	0.7	11.9
1 cup milk	87	8.5	0.2	12.4
1 peach	38	0.6	0.1	9.7
	547	40.6g.	26.1g.	48.1g.

And these are just the final figures. To arrive at them was a juggling act that took the two of us arithmetical idiots about six pages of scrawling and scratching. And often we erred. I recall once that I added when I should have subtracted (or was it the other way around?) and my dinner worked out twenty grams short of carbohydrates; so I added a hunk of French bread and a mound of peas for which I had absolutely no desire. When I refigured afterwards, because I was puzzled at having ended up so far off, it turned out that instead of being twenty grams short, the additional stuffing had made me about forty grams over, and as a result I spilled like Niagara Falls.

It wasn't long before I realized why the exchange lists had been invented. What was the advantage of eating a greater variety of foods if your stomach was always tied in mathematical knots over it? Barbara, who is possibly even slightly worse as a mathematician than I, was torn asunder between wanting me to join her in exotic dining and hating the pre-meal arithmetic lesson. From inspiration born of frustration she evolved another of her famous theories: Why bother counting all those proteins and fats and calories, if it's only the carbohydrates that do a diabetic damage? I had to admit that, since I had no weight problem—or, rather, that I had an inverse weight problem—the extra calories I might consume on a non-counted diet wouldn't hurt. But at this stage of my diabetic development I was strictly party line and I resisted Barbara's revisionist theories.

To convince me she called the Kremlin, that is, the local affiliate chapter of the American Diabetes Association, and put the question to them: "Is it only the carbohydrates that make a diabetic spill?" She got an affirmative. As you can see, it was the way she phrased her question that got her the answer she wanted. I'm sure the answer would have been more than somewhat different had she made her inquiry honestly, as, "I have this diabetic friend who wants to eat unusual foods that aren't on the exchange lists, but she and I are getting tired of figuring the nutritional value of everything she eats; so would it be all right if we just counted the carbohydrates and forgot about the proteins and fats and calories?" Then, I'm sure, the answer would have been that I should follow the proper nutritionally balanced diet my doctor had prescribed and consult him if I wanted to make any changes.

Barbara's count-the-carbohydrates-only theory, however, was not as bizarre as it sounded to me in those early diabetic days. Our later research has revealed that it is the diet method recommended for underweight and normal-weight diabetics by the British, French, and Australian diabetic associations. The French make a very blunt distinction between what they call the "thin" (*maigre*) diabetics and the "fat" (*gras*) diabetics. The "fat" ones only are put on the traditional weighed and calorie-controlled diet, in order to shed some pounds.

I experimented with this carbohydrate-only theory for about a week and, as far as I could tell, it worked beautifully. I found I could hold my meal counts in my head when I was dealing with a single set of figures. I didn't spill, and since my carbohydrate needs were being met, I didn't reel off in the other direction either. With evidence of a week's achievement to back up my question, I broached it to my doctor on my next visit. (It was No. 2 doctor.) He didn't recoil in horror at all. He only advised me that if I ate more than the prescribed amount of fats, I should make them the nonhydrogenated variety for the sake of my cardiovascular system.

Ever since then I've used this calculate-the-carbohydrates-only method of eating, and not only have I fared well at the table, while keeping my blood sugar down, but my doctor is so impressed with my carbohydrate memory bank that often he compliments me on what he calls my "mastery of the diet." And while what I have painted here may seem a rather impressionistic diet on the surface, when you look at the total picture, it is almost classically balanced. I have learned which foods fit into which exchange groups, and I make it a point to eat an appropriate amount of food from each group at each meal, because I realize that one of the objectives of the exchange diet is to insure that foods essential to good health are eaten in their proper proportions.

Now, while I don't adhere to the exchange lists in the strictest sense, I can see their advantage for those who are overweight and must control their calories and for those who, for varying reasons, prefer an easy-to-follow diet. The exchange system allows you to eat properly without bothering to learn the principles of nutrition or even to memorize the carbohydrate content of foods. My newly diabeticized colleague at the college accepted his exchange list diet without a quibble and has never strayed from it or, it seems, even had a desire to. Once I told him ecstatically that we had just received an analysis of Carlsberg beer and that it had only 5.6 grams of carbohydrate, 4.4 less than any other beer. He looked at me blankly and said, "What's a carbohydrate?"

But even those people who prefer to stick totally to the exchange-list system don't have to be as deprived of variety as they have been, for recently a woman in Northridge, California, Mrs. T. W. Vaught, went to work on the lists and expanded them. Mrs. Vaught is the mother of a great medical rarity, identical twin daughters only one of whom has diabetes. Wanting her diabetic daughter to lead the proverbial normal life that diabetes books are always advertising, she tried to make this more nearly possible by converting a vast number of additional foods into exchange list equivalents. Naturally, her amplifications are slightly tot-skewed, featuring treats such as popsicles and marshmallows. There is, however, also much on her lists for the venturesome adult eater. Any list that has caviar, frog legs, and two-finger poi has to be a remarkable breakthrough.

Mrs. Vaught has an additional theory on diabetic diets. She doesn't believe in "dietetic foods." She would rather bake and calculate the exchange equivalents of regular cookies and cakes than use the special low-cal products and recipes. Her only concession is artificial sweetener for dishes like custards and cereal.

I personally find the low-calorie and sugarless products a great boon to diabetic diets. Indeed, if one has to have diabetes, there's no better place or time to have it than in the U.S.A. in the last third of the twentieth century. When else and where else could you find such a varied assortment of artificially sweetened products on the shelves of your neighborhood market? I use almost all of them from time to time. I chew sugarless gum, drink low-cal soft drinks, smear a bit of artificially sweetened jam on my breakfast toast, lightly drizzle artificially sweetened syrup on my occasional pancakes and waffles and French toast, have a piece of dietetic chocolate now and then, and stir up dietetic puddings and gelatin desserts when the fruit selection in the market is poor.

There are a lot of scare articles these days on cyclamates—the sugar substitutes that have taken over from saccharin in recent years—saying that they have harmful side-effects if used in excess. But then, almost anything has harmful side-effects if used in excess. I use these artificially sweetened products only as much as I did their sugarful counterparts in my pre-diabetic days, which wasn't ever excessive.

As for those recipes from diabetic cookbooks and newsletters for diabetics, though I realize that they're great menu-enhancers if you must keep strict account of calories and exchange equivalents, I've given them up and gone back to my good collection of gourmet cookbooks—*Gourmet,* Volumes 1 and 2; the Chamberlains' *Flavor of France;* Julia Child's two volumes; *The New York Times Cookbook;* and so on. It's astonishing how many *haute cuisine* recipes are ideal for diabetics—veal scaloppine alla Marsala, beef stroganoff, bouillabaisse, scampi, lamb and chicken curries, shish kebab.

Now, lest you've gained the impression that I've gradually reverted to my former gourmet style of dining and that I've circumvented the diabetic regime, I want to say forthrightly that this is not true. My menus are vastly different from what they were before that March 17. I eat *more* good meals now, not only because I eat a good meal every time I sit down at the table, but also because I eat a greater variety of foods. Barbara, in fact, has noticed a great change for the better in my dining habits, and I admit to it. I used to be a fussy eater. There was a long list of foods I refused to touch at all, and now only cucumbers are in that category. I used to pick over my plate like a spoiled cat, nudging the serving askew and never finishing an entire portion of anything. Now I tie into my food with relish and not a crumb is left when I put down my fork. It's most satisfying to the cook, and it's the best medicine my diabetes could have.

But, stay, I mustn't end this dining chapter quite yet. There is still one vital question I haven't answered. What about truffles? Have they ever come back into my life? We wrote to the Department of Agriculture for an analysis and this was our answer:

We consider the meager data we have inadequate for supplying the composition values for truffles. Winton, A. L., and Winton, K. B., in "The Structure and Composition of Foods," John Wiley and Sons, Inc., 1935, cited work done in 1889, but the interpretation of the data for carbohydrate is in doubt.

So, apparently, nobody *does* know the truffles I've seen, as far as their nutritional analysis is concerned. But at $3.00 an ounce, I think I could safely advise a diabetic to feel free to eat all the truffles anybody ever offers him. That's what I plan to do.

Chapter 6

EATING OUT
OF HOUSE AND HOME

So far you've heard only half the story, the half that has to do with eating safely at home. What do we diabetics do when we go out into the world of restaurants to seek our fortunes— or misfortunes?

My initial decision about restaurant dining was that I could eat out successfully only if I went to Very Expensive French Restaurants. Since I once took cooking lessons at the Cordon Bleu in Paris, the ingredients of French dishes are no mystery to me. And the traditional French restaurant menu looks as if it had been devised by the French Diabetic Association. There are always plenty of fresh vegetables, and a fruit and cheese dessert is always available. In the best French restaurants everything is à la carte, so that you don't have to nudge piles of unwanted carbohydrate around your plate and feel that you're wasting food when there are people all over the world who don't have enough to eat. (I am of the generation whose mothers were always hounding them with tragic tales of the starving children of someplace-or-other in order to get them to clean their plates, and it has left its psychic mark.)

Think how lovely it would have been if I could have perpetuated for the rest of my life this little fraud about being able to eat only in Very Expensive French Restaurants. But early on I gave it up, and once you pass through the door of other restaurants, you can't go home again. In the first place, I was forced to acknowledge that on a single isolated evening most of us diabetics can eat anywhere and get away with it. Yes, even in those ghastly establishments whose idea of a salad is carrot scrapings in orange jello and whose idea of a vegetable is canned or frozen succotash (2 teaspoons = 1 bread exchange; I'm planning to start a help-stamp-out-succotash movement—if you would like a bumper strip, send ten cents to the publisher for postage and handling). One unfortunate night every few months ordinarily won't do any harm. In a situation like this, just follow the inevitable-rape theory. The greatest danger for the average diabetic on insulin is not getting enough carbohydrate to keep from having a reaction, and *that,* I assure you, is the least of your worries since carbohydrate is the most obtainable of restaurant commodities.

A more serious problem for a diabetic is being on vacation, when every meal is eaten out in strange restaurants. This is also eminently copable with, and I think I have proved it. In the relatively short time since my diabetes was discovered, I've spent four weeks in Hawaii, two weeks in New York and Chicago, three weeks in Yosemite Park, a week in France, a week in Switzerland, and four days in San Francisco. Now, you may think these four days in San Francisco a rather anticlimactic trip for a Californian to mention in the more formidable company of the others, but not so. It was the greatest dining challenge of them all, because I planned it that way.

Hawaii was no problem, because I was either staying in an apartment in Waikiki, where I could fix some of my own meals alternating with carefully chosen restaurants or, even easier, selecting items from the groaning cardboard of the menus at the Hanalei Plantation on Kauai or the Hana Maui Hotel on Maui or the Mauna Kea Hotel on the Big Island.

In New York and Chicago when Barbara and I were doing book promotion, we were usually so exhausted that we had simple, easily computed fare from room service in the hotel or, when we had strength enough to go out, since we were on an expense account, we ate at—what else?—Very Expensive French Restaurants.

Our vacation in France was the easiest of them all. All the restaurants were French and, with the French attitude toward food (they spend an average of one third of their income on it), most were Very Expensive.

In the hotel where we stayed in Grindelwald, Switzerland, the Regina, the menu was extensive and the style of cooking as close as they could get to French, considering it was located in Switzerland and most of the staff was Italian.

But San Francisco. That's another story. I deliberately set that trip up to be a challenge. Or rather Barbara did. She, who is always looking for an excuse to take a trip and to eat in foreign restaurants, came up with a double play this time. Sometime during the spring semester she looked at me very seriously and said, "I'm sorry to tell you this, but we're going to have to go to San Francisco as soon as school is out."

"Why?"

"To eat."

"To eat?"

"Yes, we're going to have to eat in a different kind of foreign restaurant every meal except breakfast and see how you get along."

"Why can't we do that here in Los Angeles?"

"Because you'd be staying at home and it wouldn't be the normally abnormal life of a person on a trip." And then slightly more honestly, "Besides, the San Francisco restaurants are better than the Los Angeles ones." And then, finally, in total honesty, "Besides, I want to go to San Francisco."

When I still demurred, she looked hurt and asked if I wasn't willing to make any sacrifices for the good of our book on diabetes. As usual, I sighed and acquiesced.

Using a combination of Doris Muscatine's book *A Cook's Tour of San Francisco* and the *Holiday* Magazine Restaurant Awards list and our own remembrances of restaurants past, we plotted our eating course. Our final list contained this selection of restaurants:

1 Chinese
1 German
1 Italian
1 old-style San Francisco
1 Indian

1 Greek
1 uniquely San Francisco sandwich dispensary
1 "elegant setting for lunch"

Although I begged for just one French restaurant, Barbara was firm in her refusal, citing the truth that we had already proved those beyond all doubt, both in France itself and right here at home in Sherman Oaks, where we're always popping around the corner to what we like to think of as our local bistro, Jean's Blue Room, for a guaranteed spill-free repast.

Although Barbara begged for just one Japanese restaurant, I was firm in *my* refusal. The Japanese staple, sukiyaki, is always made with unknown quantities of sugar and/or sweet wine. Tempura, with its batter coating, wipes out bread exchanges or, in my case, carbohydrate allowances, in a hurry. Rice is more of the same. I'm allergic to cucumbers, which Japanese restaurants like to feature in their salads. And, to be honest, I just don't care for Japanese foods. Actually, a diabetic could do very well with one Japanese dish, mizutaki, which is chunks of beef or chicken cooked at the table in broth. And, naturally, if you have the taste for it, you could eat as much sashimi (raw fish) as you wanted. Sukiyaki, too, if you made it at home using artificial sweetener instead of sugar, would be excellent, and even I, a Japanese-cuisine-ophobe, admit it's delicious.

We began our dining-in-restaurants research project the night before we actually took off for San Francisco, because we wanted to add a Mexican restaurant to our list. Since there's a very good one, the Casa Vega, just a block from my apartment, we thought it would be foolish to hike all over the hills of San Francisco looking for one.

I approached this meal with particular trepidation. Early in my diabetes career, when I didn't know a carbohydrate from a protein, I had really had a spill-a-thon as a result of dining in this neighborhood restaurant, and I hadn't returned since, nor had I been to any other Mexican restaurant. This time I ordered carefully, determined to eat exactly the forty grams of carbohydrate I allow myself at dinner.

Menu-at-a-Glance

Salad with oil and vinegar dressing
Chicken taco
Beef enchilada
Chiles rellenos
Carta Blanca draft beer
5 tortilla chips

I evaluated the five tortilla chips like five potato chips (1 carbohydrate each = 5). Since the tortillas in the taco and the enchilada have the combined carbohydrate value of only two-thirds of a piece of bread, I figured they would give me ten grams of carbohydrates. Ten more would take care of the sauce and miscellaneous items. I knew I'd get at least five in the vegetables of the salad and the taco filling and the chile of the chile relleno. I skipped dessert, deciding I'd used up those ten carbohydrates with the beer.

I've never enjoyed a Mexican dinner as much. Probably the feeling that I was doing something wild contributed to my enjoyment. But, nevertheless, it was delicious and pleasantly filling, although afterward I didn't feel leaden-stomached as I used to in nondiabetic days gone by, when, instead of the chile relleno, I would have downed two or three tortillas smeared with butter and wrapped around refried beans.

Score: no fits, no spills, and therefore no errors. I still was able even after all this to have my usual before-bed milk and graham cracker, with no spilling problem then, either.

The next day we took the two o'clock flight from Hollywood-Burbank airport to San Francisco. Now, on these San Francisco meals I'm not going to count out each carbohydrate, because, to be honest, I can't. I guessed a lot. There has to be some amount of guesswork in the diabetic eating biz, even if you're on the exchange lists, unless, of course, you want to be like the Englishman described by Iris Holland Rogers in *Social Problems of the Diabetic*: ". . . A man on the railway, who had had seven ounces of onion every night for 12 years, wondered if it would be safe to have a bit of a change, his wife complained so of her daily cry over peeling them."

So rather than this, I take a chance. And here's my guesswork schedule and what it wrought in those five days.

First Day—Dinner—The Shadows (German)

Menu-at-a-Glance

¼ cup lentil soup
Lettuce and tomato salad with creamy
    French dressing
½ cup sauerkraut
½ cup purée of pea
2 smoked pork loin chops with sauce
5 ounces German beer
1 cube vanilla ice cream

We decided to start off with what should be a hard one. Although I often eat knockwurst or bratwurst and sauerkraut at home—it's a fine diabetic combination—tonight I was going to try for a non-sausage repast. Barbara nudged me toward the Kassler Rippchen (smoked pork loin) rather then the sauerbraten she selected for herself, because the former came with sauerkraut, while the latter burdened the carbohydrate scales with potato pancakes.

All in all, I would have been better off sticking to the sausage route, even though I craved something a little more dramatic, because the Kassler Rippchen was covered with a thick red-brown sauce, which, since I knew not what it contained, I had to mostly scrape aside. It was also somewhat saddening to be able to have only one-fourth of a very small cup of the soup, since lentils are such concentrated carbohydrate pellets.

As it turned out, I could have eaten more than I did, because after dinner we made what seemed like an uphill-all-the-way hike from the restaurant to the Coit Tower to the Fairmont Hotel. There, I was so worried that I had used up all my carbohydrates that I made myself drink a brandy and Benedictine to replenish the supply (about six grams). Another walk of two blocks to our hotel, a slug of milk, and so to bed.

Second Day—Breakfast—Sears

Menu-at-a-Glance

½ grapefruit
1 egg
3 strips bacon
1 slice French toast
1 teaspoon dietetic jam
Coffee

Sears is our favorite San Francisco breakfast spot. Their specialties are eighteen dollar-size Swedish pancakes and French toast made with San Francisco sourdough bread. Here we usually divide an order of one or the other, or Barbara orders and gives me enough to equal the carbohydrates I would normally consume in toast.

This morning Barbara gave me some of her French toast. I ate it with some diabetic jam I had brought along. To Barbara's disgust, I had left my dietetic syrup at home, considering it just too much junk to drag along. She kept muttering about how French toast was only good with syrup. Then she got an idea. "Say, maybe they keep a bottle of dietetic syrup here for people on diets."

"I doubt it. People with good sense who are on diets usually don't tempt themselves by frequenting pancake places."

But on the way out she asked the owner-cashier. And indeed they did. Moral: always ask. You never know which places will be so considerate as to supply diabetic needs and which others may become considerate if they're asked often enough.

Since breakfast is hardly ever a problem for a diabetic, I won't go over my daily fruit, egg, bacon, and pancake or French toast ration for the rest of the San Francisco stay.

Second day—Morning Snack

This is another one I won't repeat for each day. In San Francisco we always stay in a hotel where not only are the room rates remarkably low, but they include a free continental breakfast of orange juice, doughnut, and coffee, which they deliver to the room on request. What we do is go out for an early breakfast, then return to our luxurious room overlooking the back windows of the Elizabeth Arden salon and write until about noon, using the continental breakfast as a mid-morning coffee break. I eat the doughnut and hide the orange juice in the medicine chest as an emergency fit preventative.

Second Day—Lunch—Empress of China

Menu-at-a-Glance

> Chicken with mushrooms (½ order)
> Imperial beef (½ order)
> ½ cup rice
> Fortune cookie

Here's another diabetic truth that is a gastronomic joy and a financial tragedy. Very Expensive Chinese Restaurants are about as good for the diabetic as Very Expensive French ones. That isn't too surprising, since the Chinese cuisine ranks along with the French as one of the two greatest in the world, and fully as much thought and research has gone into its development and refinement. The Very Expensive assures that instead of getting an infinitesimal morsel of pork lost in a lump of fried batter and covered with canned pineapple, you receive something more like what I got at the Empress of China.

As for their chicken with mushrooms, all I can say is, wow, what mushrooms! Three different vareties, including my favorite, the big black flavorful ones. The Imperial beef was slices of beef so tender they might have been from beer-fed and gin-rubbed cattle, such as they have in Japan, in a delectable sauce that had much less cornstarch in it than in the less Very Expensive Chinese Restaurants, and lots and lots of crispy, unlimp Chinese vegetables, the majority of which are of the "A" variety, diabetically speaking.

We ordered à la carte, because on the luncheon special along with the Imperial beef there was a sweet and sour something-or-other which I considered too risky. Barbara has been grumbling at herself ever since, because, although the menu said firmly, "No substitutions," she felt she should have tried anyway. Not only would our lunch have cost us less, as luncheon specials do, but we would have also had a cup of soup, which, considering the quality of the rest of the dishes, must have been a wonder.

Barbara's reason for not asking was that our waiter spoke mainly Chinese, one of the few languages in which she doesn't know how to say "diabetic." One of us probably should have given it a try, though. I'm sure we will in such cases in the future. After all, the worst they can say is no, and people hardly ever say no to a reasonable request from a diabetic.

After the luncheon, another walk from Grant Street to Market and Montgomery. This was a good deal farther than either of us wanted to walk in the city-gritty wind off the Bay. We had planned to go to the library to do some research, but Market Street was all torn up with subway construction. The buses and streetcars which normally ran there were doing odd deviations. There were also no cabs that we could find, because the airport bus system was on strike and most of the cabs were off engaged in the more lucrative air-passenger toting occupation. In order to make it on hoof back to the hotel from Market Street (uphill, of course), I had to stop at David's delicatessen and eat three-fourths of a bagel and butter with a cup of tea.

Second Day—Dinner—L'Odeon (Greek)

Menu-at-a-Glance

Chef's mixed green salad
1 piece San Francisco bread
Moussaka (eggplant and lamb)
⅙ Crenshaw melon

Another small contretemps here. Since we had had an exotic lunch, it was our plan to go to the Fly Trap, which was listed in *A Cook's Tour of San Francisco* as one of the better San Francisco-style restaurants, where we could get food that was a little more on the normal side, such as fish or veal not too sauced up. After we finally managed to capture one of the elusive cabs, we gave the driver the name of the restaurant and its address. He turned around to inspect us. "Ladies, how long has it been since you were in San Francisco?"

"Oh, about a year."

"Well, the Fly Trap's been torn down for a year and a half and there's a high-rise office building there now."

Since fitting time was drawing nigh, we didn't have time to ponder our selection. We just shot him the first restaurant name from our list that came to mind, L'Odeon, a Greek establishment.

I immediately began to, in Barbara's term, "sour over." I wasn't happy to be having to eat so flamboyantly twice in one day, and obviously my blood sugar was sinking slowly in the West, because I began to manifest my hypoglycemic stubbornness in refusing to do what was good for me.

Barbara did manage to get me to order a manhattan rather than a martini, but the sweet vermouth in this cocktail only delivers about seven carbohydrates, hardly enough to throw a life preserver to the blood sugar.

Right before me there on the table was a basket of San Francisco sourdough bread, which is in my opinion one of the world's great breads. Normally, I would eagerly consume all my diet would allow any time, any place. But now I wouldn't touch it, delivering one of my favorite pre-dinner lines: "I don't want to stuff myself with bread and not enjoy the meal." Stuffing, of course, was not what Barbara was pushing for, as she later pointed out, just a half-piece to keep me sane. Naturally, I wouldn't have anything to do with the maraschino cherry in my manhattan, either, fishing it out as if it were a dead fly.

There was listed on the menu an interesting-looking Greek salad that had cheese and such in it, but since one of the "and suches" mentioned was cucumbers, although Barbara urged me to order it, I refused. She offered to ask them to leave out the cucumbers, but I wouldn't let her, because (and here's another of my classic hypoglycemic lines) "I'm sick and tired of always making scenes in restaurants." She ordered the Greek salad for herself. It looked marvelous and, incidentally, had no cucumbers in it that night, and I had a comparatively dull mixed green.

My main dinner selection was moussaka, which is a lamb and eggplant casserole. It was very good, I know, but I didn't enjoy it much, because by this time Barbara had soured over, too (it's very catching), and we just grimly chewed without any pleasant dinner-table conversation. She did break the silence long enough to point out that I was hardly eating any carbohydrate, since the salad and moussaka both contained almost zero. I sullenly played with about a half of a piece of bread.

I was lucky to get the Crenshaw melon for dessert. The waiter was very doubtful that he could find any fruit in the kitchen. They favored rich Greek pastries.

Obviously, I didn't spill on this dinner. In fact, back at the hotel I had to drink an extra big glass of milk and eat two graham crackers in order to feel certain I could get through the night without having a mild reaction in my sleep.

Third Day—Lunch—Tommy's Joynt

Menu-at-a-Glance

Round of beef sandwich on roll
1 cup coleslaw
1 stein steam beer
½ large apple

A good night's sleep and my breakfast pancake ration made me human again. I was ready for a pleasant lunch, and I got it. San Francisco has a number of these buffet-like dispensaries, places where you can get marvelous French-dip beef, pork, ham, or barbecue sandwiches, salads, and plate lunches du jour, such as turkey legs, short ribs, and sausages. The kind of food they offer is what I would imagine to be like the free lunches in one of the more swinging turn-of-the-century saloons. I would like to pay special tribute to Tommy's Joynt, because, *annus mirabilis,* they have a large, complete fruit basket. I chose a big crunchy apple, ate half of it for dessert, and saved the other half for an afternoon snack.

Our after-lunch exercise was walking to the Civic Center and visiting the San Francisco art gallery and doing some research in the library.

Third Day—Dinner—Fior d'Italia (*Italian*)

Menu-at-a-Glance

Mixed green salad
Antipasto: pâté, ricotta, shrimp, vegetables
2 ravioli
Chicken Fior (with mushrooms and artichokes)
1 piece San Francisco bread
Strawberries (5 giant)

Nothing special happened here, except that I didn't turn into a Mrs. Hyde from low blood sugar.

Another mighty walk after dinner from around the Coit Tower to the Top of the Mark and then home again to our more humble digs and my usual bedtime milk.

Fourth Day—Lunch—Bardelli's (*old-style San Francisco*)

Menu-at-a-Glance

Mixed green salad
Grilled sole
1 piece San Francisco bread
Strawberries (10 medium)

Well, I did it again, only more so. I decided that since it was downhill all the way—about six blocks—from our hotel to the restaurant and since the cable cars that made the run were oozing tourists, I would walk it, even though it was already lunch time for me, before we even left the room.

I made the walk all right, but when we got to the restaurant, we found a pack of would-be lunchers milling inside the door.

We didn't know of any other place close enough to go to, and we knew that with the current cab problem we couldn't possibly find one to take us to a farther-away restaurant. There was nothing to do but wait it out. As an added nicety, a burly man who came in after us pushed ahead of Barbara and gave his name for a table for two; so we were even further behind.

We sat down in the little anteroom off the bar. A waitress approached and asked if we would like a cocktail.

"No," I answered.

"Don't you think it would be a good idea if you had a Bloody Mary?" Barbara asked in her best horse-gentling voice.

"No!"

Barbara shook her head sadly, and the waitress moved on. I just sat there with my face hard, while Barbara tried to cheer me along with promises of food just around the corner. I was not to be cheered. In fact, I began an irate tirade about how awful it is to try to get a meal in a restaurant and how they're all terrible and why was I here when I could be home and happy.

This sort of talk always gets to Barbara more than anything else I can say. Ever since I found I have diabetes she has lived in mortal dread that I will let it turn me into a house-bound recluse and she will lose her most available and fairly well-broken-in travel companion.

So this prompted her to launch into a tirade on how you *have* to eat out when you travel, and travel is well worth the inconveniences, and you have to expect the unexpected, and come on, *please* have a Bloody Mary or a screwdriver or just plain juice, if you like, and if you aren't careful you're going to make yourself into an invalid who just never leaves the house and always eats exactly seven ounces of onions for dinner like the Englishman and never does anything exciting.

"That's just exactly what I'm going to make myself into and right now!" I stood up and strode out the door.

Barbara galloped after me. "What are you doing? Where are you going?" she said, running along beside me.

"Home."

"Home? You don't mean home to Los Angeles, do you?"

"Yes."

"How are you going to get there? Are you going to walk?"

"I guess so."

Barbara was tugging at my arm, begging me to come back to the restaurant, looking about ready to burst into tears of one kind or other.

"You can't walk all the way home. You'll go into shock. In fact, you must already be in it." Barbara said it was like trying to reason with a lunatic.

But after striding one long block, crossing one busy intersection, and going on another half-block, I ran out of steam and allowed myself to be pulled back to the restaurant and given a Bloody Mary, while Barbara went to the maître d' and got our names back on the waiting list, explaining that we had had to go out and meet someone for a minute.

I perked up right away. It's always like dropping a coin into a jukebox—instant pleasant music. It was, incidental'y, the tastiest Bloody Mary I've ever had. I don't know why I resisted it.

I didn't order lunch exactly brilliantly, though, because the menu said grilled sole and I didn't realize it would be like fried sole and have a carbohydrous coating that I had to scrape off, unless I wanted to skip bread, which I certainly didn't in San Francisco. Barbara offered to trade me her braised oxtails, but I declined because I was really in the mood for fish. I did let her pick out her carrots and pieces of celery to give me some of the vegetables which I feel I can't get through a meal without these days. I ordered a bowl of big, fat, sweet northern California strawberries for dessert. I could only eat half the portion and gave Barbara the rest. Reward enough, I hoped, for her having to play her pre-prandial role of matron at Bedlam.

What we learned, among other things, from this encounter was that if you're playing it close to the wire and you think blood sugar is running out, it might be wise to inform the maître d' of the fact. If he is at all a reasonable human being, as most of them are, he should be willing and able to sneak you in ahead of the non-problem children, who would have no way of knowing you didn't have a prior reservation. At least it's worth a try.

Fourth Day—Dinner—India House (Indian)

Menu-at-a-Glance

Mixed green salad
Chicken curry with rice
1 chapatti
8-ounce bottle of beer
20 grapes (Thompson seedless)

We started with a cocktail. I had to have one of my uncomplex usuals. Barbara got to indulge in a Pimm's Cup No. 1 (the gin variety). The only thing that saved me from coveting her frosted silver mug and unusual libation was that the garnish of a Pimm's Cup No. 1 is that old devil cucumber.

In my dinner ordering I had a preconceived notion that I wanted chicken curry. Bad move. I couldn't eat enough of the accompanying garnishes (sambals) to make it worthwhile, because they included raw onions, which I don't like, and raisins, sweet pickle relish, sweetened coconut, and chutney, which I can't very well eat if I want to eat anything else with carbohydrates.

(A diabetic can, by the way, easily have curry at home by picking the sambals with care, as we point out in the recipe in Part Two. Sliced tomatoes, ground peanuts, grated eggs, bacon, sliced green peppers, dill pickles, dried fish are all perfect and perfectly diabetically acceptable. Australia even produces a kind of sugar-free chutney which would be worth digging around an import shop to try to find.)

In addition, although I started with a salad, I still felt undervegetabled. What I should have selected, Barbara and I decided later, was the kebabs and curried vegetables. (See Part Two.) Since I had a chapatti (unleavened Indian bread) with my salad, I couldn't eat much rice with my curry. For mouth-cooling purposes, I had a bottle of beer. Barbara, lucky, healthy-pancreas-ed wretch, stuck with Pimm's Cups.

She, by the way, enjoyed her meal immensely, but told me later she would have enjoyed it more had I not been complaining all through it. It would be nice if we diabetics could learn to put a good face on, even when we're not quite delighted with the food we've selected in a restaurant. It does, I know, rather spoil things for others when we spread our wet crying towels across the dinner table, and it doesn't really do us any particular good. No, we should just determine to do better next time and strike it up to experience, which is, as Oscar Wilde said, the name we give to our mistakes.

Fifth Day—Lunch—Redwood Room, Clift Hotel

Menu-at-a-Glance

1 large Bloody Mary
1 piece sautéed halibut
Melba toast
Green beans
½ serving of raspberries

San Francisco followed the old show-business edict, "Always leave 'em laughing." The Redwood Room was, indeed, as Doris Muscatine called it, an "elegant setting for lunch," and the meal was just right for me both as a food lover and as a diabetic. The Bloody Mary was so large (in the juice sense of it) that I was able to use it in lieu of a salad. My sautéed halibut was so fresh it must have been frolicking under the Golden Gate that very A.M., and the accompanying green beans vied with the fish for freshness. I had a piece of melba toast for carbohydrate ballast and for dessert half of a serving of fresh raspberries, which I had been hungrily eyeing in all the little markets tucked in under apartment buildings on the ascent to Nob Hill, but which I had never until this time found on a restaurant menu.

Home again somewhat wiser than when I left. What had I learned? On the negative side, I learned not to play it too close at eating time. There seems to be an ironical rule in diabetic dining that if you start out late—or almost late—you're going to encounter delays every step along the way and wind up in fitting territory. While if you allow yourself more than enough time, things will go off without a hitch and you'll wind up eating earlier than you really want to. But if this be your choice, it's no choice at all. Always go for the early dinner for the sake of your health and the sanity of your friends, and you'll have the dividend of finding the restaurant less crowded and noisy.

Another reason you should eat a little earlier than usual when you're on a vacation is that you're getting more exercise than normal. Sightseeing and walking a lot as I was, it was rather hard to tell exactly how much of my carbohydrate I'd used up and when. Incidentally, because of this extra exercise you can usually eat more on a vacation than you do at home. This is pretty nice, since this is exactly when you want to eat more.

On the positive learning side, I confirmed what I already suspected—a diabetic can eat out in restaurants for extended periods without great risk of spilling and can eat a vast assortment of varied viands. All the diabetic has to do in restaurants—or at home—is know what he's doing.

Chapter 7

PUBLIC DIABETIC, PRIVATE DIABETIC

There are two schools, the public and the private, in which the diabetic learns his lessons—his diabetic three R's. These three R's, according to diabetic manuals, are Regulation, Regularity, and Routine. From what I've learned so far in diabetic kindergarten and first grade, though, I would say there are another three R's a diabetic's likely to become familiar with— Rule-breaking, Risk-taking, and Reactions.

This is particularly true for the Public Diabetic. I hardly had time to take stock of the fact that I was a diabetic before I had to go public with it. Our firstborn book, *Alice in Womanland*, was due to toddle off the press only three months after my diagnosis. Now, having a book published hardly makes you an instant celebrity like a rock-and-roll singer or a heart-transplant surgeon, but it does demand appearances on radio and television programs. That's how books are promoted these days.

As Joyce Lubold pointed out in her funny but painfully true article about book promotion in *Publisher's Weekly*, what the author needs to be, in such a situation, is "an aggressive, nimble-tongued huckster . . . a glad-handing stand-up comic," but what he's more likely to be is "a pock-faced introvert working obscurely somewhere in a garret . . . a naive, shy, stumble-footed type, all tangled up in his own inhibitions."

Barbara and I were no exception to the reticent-writer rule. Both of us found our marrow turning to gelatin and our minds to cream of wheat at even the thought of a camera or a microphone. In fact, after publication day, when the Los Angeles "Promotion in Motion" firm that was assigned to sock us into the public eye called to inform us of our bookings, we in our terror refused one after another. After several negative exchanges, the frustrated PR man put it to us squarely. "Come on now, girls. What's the bit? You got something you're trying to hide? Level with me. Is it a police record or what?"

Finally, telling ourselves that we were being silly, we clenched our rattling teeth and gradually let them break us in with a few local Los Angeles appearances: Ron McCoy, Louis Lomax, Keene at Noon, Feature Page with Ted Meyers, and a show called Moss and Thurman, which was—we trust, not significantly —canceled by the station the night after we appeared on it.

My diabetes wasn't disturbed by any of these performances, because they were scattered, with several days between each for R & R (Rest and Recuperation), as they put it for front-line fighters. When we were flown to San Francisco, however, it was a different and less slow-paced story. We had to struggle through a full three-day schedule of three TV shows, five radio programs, a newspaper interview, and a huge cocktail-autographing party at the American Library Association convention with a late, late dinner afterward. (Diabetic rule: Do not delay meals.) I was on Tolinase at the time and my main worry was spilling (which I didn't), plus, of course, totally exhausting myself (which I did). (Diabetic rule: Do not get overly tired.)

After the San Francisco workouts we were called back for a week of promotion in New York and Chicago. We prepared for the ordeal by spending a couple of weeks in Hawaii to put a little color in our pock faces and strength in our stumbling feet. We might as well have stayed in our respective garrets, because all of our vitality and color were drained off in the first day in New York. You really can't blame a publisher for getting as much mileage as possible out of authors. After all, it does cost a number of dollars to haul them cross-country and pay for their hotel room and dinners in Very Expensive French Restaurants. So they got their mileage out of us and, to be honest, we compounded the felony by deviously setting up meetings with other New York publishers in the little spare time we had.

Another problem for us was that all of our appearances were booked in advance without our knowledge and without our having any veto power at all. One look at the prearranged bookings and we were terrorized. Our first appearance was with Alan Burke. That was like trying to climb Everest before you even get your boots laced. Luckily for me and my nervous system, Barbara and I had early in the game hit upon a ruse that spared me somewhat. We discovered that the person who sits closest to Mr. Interlocutor is the one who gets asked most of the questions. This is especially true of TV, where in the camera's eye three's a crowd, and it prefers to focus on two having their intimate exchange of "ideas." When I was feeling spent, which was about 85 percent of the time in those days, Barbara would put herself next to the interviewer, where she could do most of the talking. She complained that she created the impression of being a babbling publicity hound, but I maintained that that was no worse than my appearing to be the tongue-tied village idiot.

As we were plunked into our swivel chairs under the hot lights of Alan Burke's stage, both our systems were awash with adrenalin. (Diabetic rule: Avoid nervous tension.) Like most things you dread, however, the anticipation far exceeded the actuality. Because Mr. Burke was such a gracious host, we felt at ease.

Since I had used up all my juices in the worry warm-up, though, I had to just sit there something like a waxworks figure, even when a member of the studio audience directly addressed a question to me. I don't remember much of what happened and neither does Barbara, although she fuzzily recalls rattling off patently stupid answers to the audience's questions about their marital difficulties, with the somber air of authority of a Margaret Mead. Although our book is a satirical treatment of the woman question and makes fun of all the advice-mongers, on television and radio we often found ourselves coming on like sociologists rather than humor writers.

On to Chicago, where we were placed in the hands of a truly remarkable publicity woman, the aptly named Dorothy Strong. She had unlimited energy and enthusiasm and assumed we had the same. She also had unlimited radio/TV contacts. Consequently, our three days with her contained as much action as all our Los Angeles, San Francisco, and New York performances put together. How's this for a one-day schedule?

7:00–9:00 A.M.   The Morning Show
10:50 A.M.   Martha Crane Show
11:30 A.M.–12:30 P.M.   Autographing at Marshall Field & Co. and at Kroch's and Brentano's
4:30–6:30 P.M.   Tom Duggan Show
7:00–8:00 P.M.   Del Clark Show
11:00 P.M.–1:30 A.M.   Jack Eigen Show

Even the least knowledgeable newly hatched diabetic can see an early basic flaw in this program. That is, when does one eat breakfast? Neither the hotel coffee shop nor room service functioned before 7:00 A.M., and we were to report to the studio at 6:00 A.M. Even though with the oral drugs hypoglycemia was a minor consideration, I knew I couldn't plow through the morning with nothing inside me without risking drifting into more than my customary television vagueness. But Dorothy Strong, with her typical energy and enthusiasm, volunteered to get up in what would be the middle of the night and fix something for me and bring it along.

The next morning she arrived with coffee, toasted buttered English muffins (foil-wrapped and still warm), and a can of orange juice. I wolfed it all down and only afterward noticed that the orange-juice can said, "Sugar added." (Diabetic rule: Avoid refined sugar.) You know the vivid green result.

This day did not end for us until 2:00 A.M. the following morning. (Diabetic rule: Maintain a schedule designed for adequate sleep and rest.)

But now that I'm on insulin, where I belong, what happens when we put on what Barbara calls our "dog and pony shows"? According to my doctor, stage fright causes the body to pump out adrenalin, which usually counteracts insulin, causing hyperglycemia (rather than hypo-). It can, however, depending on how an individual system reacts, work just the opposite, making it rather difficult to figure, to say the least.

But these dangers don't bother me anymore, since stage fright is no longer likely. In fact, now that we're on our fourth book, Barbara and I have rather turned into a couple of hams—non-sugar-cured, of course. We'd probably even be willing to do our dog and pony show on the Ed Sullivan program if called upon to do so, although that is about as likely as my eating three hot-fudge sundaes and a pecan pie for dinner tonight.

But even if you never write a book or transplant a heart or let your hair grow and take up the guitar, you still have to be a public diabetic a good deal of the time. You may have a job which involves pressures and tensions fully as great as those of TV and radio performances, and you surely go to parties and social functions, where nondiabetic food and drink are served and where there are meal delays to contend with.

In the case of dinner parties, I've found there are two approaches. These are roughly parallel to the two attitudes of Catholics when there used to be the restriction on eating meat on Fridays. One group held that if your hostess forgot and served steak or roast, you should go ahead and eat it and not waste food or be rude. The other held that you should politely decline the meat and eat everything else, hoping that the hostess would open a can of tuna or stir up an omelet for you.

I, myself, am a fence-straddler with the dining-out diet. I won't eat *everything*. I will, for example, refuse a rich dessert under most, no, I'll say *all* circumstances. But I won't stew unnecessarily, or at least not visibly, if the meal I'm presented with is a little less balanced than my usual tightrope walker or if there's a little more carbohydrate than I normally would take.

The meal delays are the real problem for a diabetic on insulin. Cocktail hours can easily become cocktail eternities, with time suspended in alcohol. Barbara cringes to recall that in the days before she knew anything about diabetes, Tom's diabetic friend Jim had come over for dinner. Tom was delayed two hours in a San Diego commuter flight tie-up. She graciously served Jim all the scotch he could want, but not even a salted peanut did she proffer, and she didn't fling the hot hors d'oeuvre into the oven until Tom arrived. She says that it was at the time very flattering to see Jim pounce upon her hors d'oeuvre offerings with such gusto, but now that she knows what she put the poor fellow through, she is sore ashamed.

When I don't know the hostess and her habits, I try to structure things in my favor ahead of time. Sometimes I take my morning injection an hour later so its full force will hit me at a so-called civilized dining hour, instead of at 5:00 or 5:30 P.M. Sometimes I eat 50–75 percent of my carbohydrate allotment before I leave home. This makes me feel much more secure, but unfortunately it can destroy the ego of my hostess, who sees me only nibbling at the periphery of her creations. As a result, I sometimes eat more than I should and spill, but not often.

There is an equation that usually works in diabetic dinner-guesting. The better the cook, the less you need to worry. A good cook usually will not put off the meal and let her *haute cuisine* run downhill while guests destroy their taste buds with alcohol. Indeed, she may serve nothing but sherry or vermouth or some such non–binge-inducing libation before dinner. And a good cook usually cooks in the French manner or some variation thereon and I've already flailed the advantages of French cooking for the diabetic.

When hostesses who are aware of my diabetes ask ahead of time what they should serve me, I always assure them that I can eat just about anything, but would appreciate a piece of fruit for dessert. If they press for more information, I will confess to them my vegetable addiction.

When I'm the hostess myself, since I'm in charge of the situation, I have no fears except for late-arriving guests, who might force me to chomp down some preventative carbohydrate, and late-staying guests, who might cause me to lose some sleep. (This latter is less a diabetic necessity than a personal early-to-bed-and-early-to-rise idiosyncrasy.)

I derive particular delight in announcing to my dinner guests that they are going to have a perfect diabetic meal and seeing them blanch and gulp at imaginings of thin gruel and barley water, then beam with surprise and delight at what they actually get. Most are especially enthralled with the vegetables, which are not so much cleverly prepared as scrupulously fresh. So effusive are they that I've begun to get the idea that a great proportion of people almost never taste a vegetable that hasn't served time in a freezer or a can. For dessert I usually serve cheese and fruit (again scrupulously fresh), but I'm not averse to making an occasional sweet-toothsome dessert soufflé or pastry for others to enjoy.

Just as by necessity I'm slightly more public than the average diabetic, I'm also by necessity slightly more private. As a divorcée, I live alone—and like it, although I had my doubts about continuing to like it after my diabetes was diagnosed, and recovering from that, my doubts doubled and trebled when I went onto insulin. Who would slip me the orange juice when I started going goofy with hypoglycemia? And even worse, I imagined myself playing the starring role in a scene like the one Bill Talbert describes in *Playing for Life:*

> I was already in a serious insulin reaction when I reached the hotel—too far gone even to remember my all-important bedtime snack. Without that buffer to protect me, I had lapsed deeper into reaction at the most hazardous time of all— while I was asleep, unaware of trouble, unable to do anything about it. Now I lay deep in its throes. . . . By the time I reached the hospital . . . I was so deep in shock that it had taken [24] hours before huge amounts of sugar solution, injected intravenously, had shown any effect.

This could happen to me, I thought, and maybe the ambulance would not come until too late. I might just lie there until I turned into a mummy. This shows how much your imagination can gallop off. In the first place, if you aren't leading the wild life Talbert was at that time, slipping off into insulin shock in the middle of the night is highly unlikely. And slipping into its opposite, diabetic coma, is almost impossible for a diabetic in good control. And even if you're in poor control, you'll get some long-range harbingers that things are amiss—thirst, hunger, excessive urination, weight loss, fatigue.

Besides, I couldn't very well mummify, because Barbara began taking it upon herself to call me early every morning—

sometimes too early for my taste—to make sure I had survived the night. And when she was out of town, she'd assign the job to a mutual friend. I find this somewhat embarrassing, but also something of a comfort; so I haven't called a halt.

Now that I'm over being plagued by living-alone fears, I have decided that, far from being a total detriment, there are actually a few advantages to being a live-alone diabetic. For one, I can take my fix sitting at the breakfast table waiting for the coffee to perk. I imagine the sight of early morning flesh-puncturing might curdle the soft-boiled eggs of most breakfast companions. Living alone, I also don't have to worry about delayed meals. I can eat whenever I want to and need to without relying on someone else to be home on time for dinner.

I find, too, that my solitary dinners now as a diabetic are more pleasant than they were before. It's a terrible temptation for a person living alone to grab something out of the refrigerator or open a can of soup, because it's just too much bother to cook a whole dinner for one person. My evening meal specialty used to be what Barbara referred to as "an avocado sandwich maybe," because every time she asked me what I was going to have for dinner I'd shrug and respond, "Oh, I don't know. Guess I'll have an avocado sandwich—maybe." Now I have my complete vege-tabled and meated and fruited dinner preceded by my regular cocktail (I prefer to still follow Dr. No. 2's "drink the same amount daily" advice). Dinner is never as dismal as in the avo-cado-sandwich-maybe days.

By necessity, with all the fruits and vegetables I eat, I've also joined Barbara in her French housewife shopping schedule—that is, going to the market almost every day. She does it, I main-tain, both because she's absent-minded and because she refuses to make a list—not, as she maintains, to get nothing but the freshest of newly arrived viands.

But these are the superficial privacies of my private life. I do have a few more private privacies. I'll begin by confessing that there are a few devious practices I apply to work my diabetes to my advantage. I know I shouldn't, but a person deserves to get some good out of the silly disease.

Not that diabetic excuses—even valid and honest ones—always work. Barbara recently tried to get me past an hour's wait at a no-reservation restaurant and was met with solid refusal. I guess that was all they could do, since the waiting room was ringed with hardset hungry faces who would no doubt have fomented a bread riot had a latecomer been slipped past them. Then, too, a young diabetic son of a friend of mine was once ripping home above and beyond the speed limit in his hot rod for dinner after a strenuous tennis game. The motorcycle policeman who stopped him was very sympathetic about the boy's impending insulin shock—as he wrote out the ticket.

And, speaking of driving, since diabetes is no excuse for committing traffic offenses and certainly is none for causing an accident, when driving I recommend following the advice of the British Diabetic Association in their pamphlet "Car Driving for Diabetics":

> The diabetic on insulin or tablets should not drive unless he has eaten a meal containing his usual carbohydrate allowance within the previous two hours. If this is not the case, the diabetic would be well advised to eat some of his carbohydrate allowance before starting his journey. He must continue to take 20 grams of carbohydrate every two hours while driving. It is always wiser to err on the side of safety.

I guess the BDA is especially conscientious about this because in England if you let yourself get hypoglycemic at the wheel, you can draw a driving-under-the-influence-of-drugs conviction. This is not illogical, because insulin *is* a drug and you *are* under its influence and you *could* do much damage in that groggy condition. It would also be wise for you to discreetly investigate to see if your state has any diabetic driving restrictions. Mine, California, examines and analyzes each case individually and usually requires a periodic report from the diabetic's doctor that all is well and that fitting is unlikely. As I say, investigate *discreetly*, though, because if you go stomping around and shouting and making a scene about it, you just might manage to get some restrictions slapped on where none exist and set diabetic freedom back twenty years. One place where your inquiries should be indiscreet, however, is with your insurance company. Make absolutely sure and certain and positive that they know you are a diabetic, and get it in writing that they know. Otherwise, in time of accident, there will be an excuse to refuse payment.

Where the law and the powers that insure are not involved, however, you can usually use your diabetes as an excuse to get away with about anything you want to, because there's such a universal, colossal ignorance concerning it. You could, for example, say, "Oh my, Agnes, I'd so like to offer to help you with the dishes, but with my diabetes I'm not allowed to handle wet things," or "Edgar, you're really very sweet and I'm quite fond of you, but I think we'd better just shake hands and say goodnight now . . . my diabetes, you know."

In such circumstances you'd probably be believed without the deceived one batting an eye. But I really prefer to base my excuses on only slightly distorted fact. There's quite enough misinformation floating around on diabetes as it is without my adding to it.

I do shamelessly use my diabetes to get my meals on time, because, all hypoglycemic hazards aside, I like to have my meals on time and always have. I use it as an excuse to go to bed early because I've always been a day rather than a night person. I use it to get out of eating at banquets, too. (If Jackie Onassis back in the days when she was Jackie Kennedy could get away without eating at them, I can, too.) I know I could easily handle the most carbohydrous of banquet fare on islolated evenings with no problem at all, but since the quality of food is usually just one millimeter this side of ghastly, if Barbara and I are speaking at a dinner gathering, I usually sigh with regret and say, "I'm so very sorry, but I'll just have to eat ahead of time. I'm on a strict diabetic diet, you know." And Barbara, playing the martyr as only she can, crumples her face and tells them that she'll forego the banquet fare, too, and eat with June because it would be cruel to make the poor thing have her meal alone.

But my all-time favorite diabetic excuse is a little more dramatic. It's based on a device for getting out of things that Barbara and I originated in *Alice in Womanland*. We call it the "Scarlet Lie": "something monumentally shocking and/or embarrassing that you make up to tell about yourself, the sort of thing you would normally tell a little white or big black lie to cover up for, the kind of statement for which there can be no response except a baffled retreat."

The ideal, all-purpose lie for a diabetic is: "Oh, my, I'd just love to but I can't. You see, that's the day I have to stay home and take my twenty-four-hour urine specimen collection."

Should you feel guilty achieving your private ends by public deception, there's a good way to salve your conscience. You can provide a public service by seeing to it that your friends and relatives are all tested for diabetes. At the risk of being considered a urine fetishist, insist when friends drop over that they test themselves, or let you test them, with your Tes-Tape or Clinitest to see if they have any danger signals.

The importance of urging your friends to take tests was brought home recently when Barbara and I, wrapped up in my diabetes as we were, let a good friend of ours, she who performs for each of us the service of weekly making domestic order out of the chaos of our respective households, advance right in front of us to the stage of diabetes at which her blood sugar was 500 and her eyesight was affected, mercifully only temporarily. All this happened without either of us recognizing she even had it. An ounce of Tes-Tape would have saved a ton of trouble for her.

Now, let's see, does that cover all of the private life of a private diabetic? I think so, although, human nature being what it is, some of you may wonder about the most publicly discussed area of private activity, sex. The husband of a friend of mine, upon learning I was taking pills for diabetes, leered and asked, "They're supposed to make you sexy, aren't they?" As usual, I was at a loss for words, although, I did come up with some brilliant ones in what the French call *l'esprit de l'escalier*. (That's thinking of a devastatingly witty response just as you're walking down the stairs leaving the party.) But from all that I've read, I don't really think that either oral compounds or insulin could be classified as aphrodisiacs. I think it's more that being an out-of-control diabetic makes you—as my friend's husband would put it—*not* sexy. This lack of interest in sex is, in fact, one of the symptoms described in *How to Live With Diabetes:*

During World War II, a young American lieutenant advancing through Germany attributed his thirst to the summer heat, and his frequent urination to the enormous quantities of beer he quaffed. But one day he became aware that his sexual urges were almost gone. This promptly brought him to the doctor and it was there that the diabetes was discovered.

If all else fails, *that* should be enough to get everyone to run out and take his blood sugar entrance examination to the diabetic school. And if a person finds he does qualify for this increasingly non-exclusive educational institution, he shouldn't, like Shakespeare's schoolboy, go creeping like a snail unwilling to school, because, although it's true that the diabetic school is no Summerhill, it doesn't have to be a sadomasochistic military academy either.

Chapter 8

GO SPILL IT
ON THE MOUNTAIN

Would you believe a diabetic skier? Of course you would. After all, you'd believe a diabetic football player like Ron Mix of USC or Coley O'Brien of Notre Dame. And Kenneth Cooper, in his book *Aerobics*, points out that skiing and football are exact equivalents in the amount of energy they consume.

All right, now that you accept a diabetic skier, would you believe a woman diabetic skier who had never been particularly athletic and who first took up skiing at the age of forty-five, two weeks after she discovered she had diabetes and who, the following year, took off on a ski holiday only three days after going onto the insulin needle? And *that* is not a snow job.

In December, three months before my D-Day, Barbara announced that she was going to give skiing a try. To me this sounded like the nuttiest idea that had come out of her since she decided to write with her left hand for a year. While it's true that she is ten years my junior, still she was four years into her brittle-boned thirties and, I felt, had no business getting herself involved in a sport so hazardous that it is grouped with prize-fighting and bobsledding as activities that are forbidden to travel guidebook writer Temple Fielding by his insurance policy.

Still, there was no talking her out of it. As she took off on her first trip to Mammoth Mountain, California, that December, I bade her farewell with the old theatrical admonition, "Break a leg!", half suspecting that she might and half hoping she would so as to snap off this lunacy before something more serious happened. But, alas, when she returned from her trip she was of healthy body. There was some doubt about her mind, though. She had one of those reverse-raccoon ski tans, and glowing from the white mask were the wild and rather frightening eyes of the True Believer. She had found Truth, Beauty, Religion. Skiing was glorious, thrilling, exhilarating, magnificent, and every other superlative in the thesaurus.

She raved on, "June, you've got to go skiing with me next time." I cringed. "We'll write articles about it. Maybe even a book. Skiing is the 'in' sport now. Editors are sobbing for ski pieces." (That's always her way of trying to con me into doing something I don't want to do.)

I told her I wouldn't be caught dead on skis. In fact, that's exactly the way I was certain I would wind up if I got on them. No. Never. Not under any circumstances would I consider going skiing. Definitely, positively, absolutely not.

And so it came to pass that in the month of February, just six weeks before my diabetes was discovered, I decided to take up skiing. Never underestimate the power of a fanatic. It wasn't entirely that she wore me down, though. It was also that I began to realize that the future of our collaboration was at stake. Margaret Mead in one of her lectures on modern marriage points out that if one of the partners is a convert to skiing and the other can't stand the sport, she doesn't hold out much hope for the union. Now, if marriage is a tenuous relationship, think how much more so a writing collaboration is. Not only are the more obvious mucilages of nuptuality nonexistent, but the only legal contract is the one for the current book, and *that* one is with the publisher and not between the collaborators.

Whenever Barbara and I were working on writing together during this period, I would see her eyes film over, and I would know that it was a case of mountain over mind. I also knew from past experience that the carrot-and-stick principle works very well with her. Although it's sometimes hard to get her to settle down to business, if you hold out a tantalizing reward, she will work like a burro to attain it. And what could be more effective than "If we finish this chapter by the end of the month, we'll go to Mammoth Mountain for a few days of skiing"? Obviously nothing. So I capitulated.

Our first trip—one to Badger Pass in Yosemite National Park—was scheduled for March 22, and you know what happened to me on March 17. But the burro had truly worked hard and deserved the promised carrot, so I packed up my new bottle of Orinase and my exchange list and away we went. Here I will confess that I cannot be credited with raw courage and rare enterprise for taking off on my first ski trip only five days after becoming a newly diagnosed diabetic. It was, in the words of Dr. Johnson, "Ignorance . . . pure ignorance."

Just like everyone else who doesn't have it (and a good many who do), I knew nothing about diabetes and the precautions a sensible diabetic should take with his bones and extremities. It was fortunate for me that the first ski trip for anyone, diabetic or not, is not a very hazardous undertaking. Most of the time is spent learning how to put on and take off the equipment. About all I did during this first excursion was sidestep up a very gentle slope and snowplow down it again in the lowest gear of the human mechanism. Still, even with my despondent mental outlook and my dietary difficulties at the Ahwahnee, I managed to come away with a heady whiff of the intoxicating ether of skiing: the grace of the skilled skier, the serenity of the slopes, and the tranquillity of being away from the nerve-cracking cacophony of the city.

As soon as we returned home, Barbara and I began our reading in depth about diabetes. We found out that moderate exercise was recommended in every book, but at the same time, though it was never stated in so many words, logic told us that stomping around in twenty pounds of equipment in the freezing cold and hurtling yourself down a mountain, every muscle tensed in terror, would not be considered a moderate form of exercise. Only walking, bowling, tennis, swimming, and other such mild sports were ever mentioned specifically. On top of that, usually the book gave a strong warning against vigorous activities concentrated in a weekend.

Then there was the whole problem of the lower extremities. We read all those admonitions about their care, especially noting:

> Be careful not to injure legs, feet, and toes.
> Do not open blisters with pins or needles.

Don't wear anything tight around your legs or ankles that
  might in any way reduce the blood supply to your feet.
Do not bathe feet in water that is too hot.
Break in new shoes gradually.
Do not wear tight or badly fitted shoes.
Do not apply adhesive tape directly to the skin.
Do not bandage feet tightly.

How could anything as sensitive as a diabetic's feet be sub-
jected to those blister-breeding grounds, those circulation-
stopping, torturous, modern-day iron boots that are frequently
so agonizing that a friend of Barbara's once remarked, "Taking
your boots off at the end of the ski day is better than sex"?

Contrary to what happened in our minds after reading about
drinking and diabetes, the more we studied the diabetic manuals,
the more we began to suspect that it might be foolhardy of me
to continue learning to ski. Even Barbara, fanatic as she was,
was worried. She later told me that in her midnight imagination
she was tortured by visions of my being hauled down the mountain on a litter by the ski patrol with a never-healing spinal fracture, or of my dying of an infected blister like President
Coolidge's son (who, incidentally, was not a diabetic).

Spring skiing closed down before we had an opportunity for
another trip, and I didn't have to face up to the issue of to ski or
not to ski until the first snows of winter. When the slope condition reports began pouring out of the radio in early November,
surprisingly there welled up within me the strangest, strongest
longing to go skiing again. In retrospect it's my opinion that at
least a part of this feeling was due to the idea that I couldn't
go, that my diabetes had slammed and locked the door on a
pleasurable activity that normal people can indulge in, that I
was, in a certain sense, an invalid.

Barbara, because of her own fears about the dangers of skiing
for me, didn't start pressuring me to join her, as I had expected
—and subconsciously hoped—she would. I knew she hadn't
abandoned the idea entirely, however, because she was quietly
engaged in a "scientific investigation" of the advisability of skiing
for diabetics. I put "scientific investigation" in quotes, because

while it is true she wrote to an outstanding, nationally known doctor for advice, whom did she choose but Merritt Stiles, former president of the U.S. Ski Association and second vice-president to the U.S. Olympic Committee, a man who had taken up skiing at the age of fifty-five and who now in his sixties skis three or four days a week from late November until late April. In other words, Barbara's writing to him was akin to someone writing to Billy Graham to ask if there might be harmful effects from a diabetic having a religious conversion.

His answer in part was:

I am no expert on diabetes, but it is my impression that most specialists in metabolic diseases recommend exercise in the treatment of diabetes. Garfield Duncan, for example, said, "Physical exercise judiciously employed by patients who have no contra-indicating conditions is of inestimable value in the treatment of diabetes. It improves the total food and carbohydrate tolerance and reduces the need for insulin." And this was back in 1947, when the profession at large was much less enthusiastic about exercise than it is at present.

. . . Your alter ego should discuss with her own physician the general advisability of exercise . . . and find out from him whether she might need to change her Tolinase dosage if she exercised actively.

A number of recent national champions in a variety of sports, including skiing, have been diabetics, which should be some comfort to your friend.

Barbara's next communiqué to Dr. Stiles was a note on the back of a Christmas card, an ecstatic, gratitude-oozing message thanking him for doubling her prospective ski time and thereby making life worth living. The entire 1967–68 ski season was still ahead, and she joyfully recounted to him our plans: four or five local trips and then in April two weeks in France and Switzerland.

For, you see, I had decided to keep on skiing. Now, Dr. Stiles' letter was hardly a carte as blanche as snow for skiing, any more than were my No. 2 doctor's words an endorsement of moderate drinking. I had, however, now decided to try a new tack with diabetes. I would assume I could do whatever I wanted to, and off-handedly I would announce it to my doctor, as if there were no possibility of my not being able to do it. As "By the way, doctor, I'll be spending the next week in Wrightwood skiing at Holiday Hill," or "Oh, say, doctor, did I mention I'm going to be flying to the Alps for a couple of weeks in April?" Since I've been working on this principle I have never once received a negative reaction from my doctor. In fact, he and his whole staff rushed through a blood sugar test for me so I could be certain everything was in order for my takeoff to France.

So in November and December I took to the ski slopes again and I was enjoying it immensely. Then shortly after Christmas I began to develop my little spilling-and-subconsciously-starving-myself problem and the Hansel and Gretel-like trail of various pills that eventually led to the needle.

In February I had to cancel one ski trip to Yosemite because the doctor wanted me in town so he could observe the reaction—or in this case non-reaction—to his latest prescription of pills. Barbara and I rescheduled our trip for two weeks later, and lo, three days before *that* one, on February 17, I had to go on the needle.

Saturday morning before the Wednesday when we were to leave for Yosemite, Barbara and I were in the doctor's office learning from Rae, the lab technician, how to give the pop. We had both assumed that the technician had diabetes, because in our blubbery society it's so rare to see a person as slender as she is that if you run across one who's associated with diabetes in any way, you immediately think he has it. As Rae was giving us the instructions, Barbara hesitantly asked if she thought it would be all right if I went ahead with our planned trip. Rae, in her customary sardonic and matter-of-fact manner, which we always enjoy and appreciate, responded, "Well, *I'm* not the doctor, but I certainly wouldn't let it stop *me*." This was a glorious go-ahead for us, thinking as we did that she was a diabetic. (We later found out she wasn't. It was just her life philosophy that you shouldn't let *anything* stop you from doing something you really want to do. Good philosophy, that, whether you're diabetic or not.)

That Monday, talking to the doctor on the telephone, I followed my casual-announcement policy and got my usual acceptance, the only caution being that I would have to cut down on my insulin or eat more because of the exercise. Since I didn't like to fiddle with the insulin dosage this early (and still don't, incidentally) and since I wanted to rediscover the wonderful world of food after my carbohydrate starvation period, I opted for eating more.

Eat more I did. In fact, I ate like six stevedores. I had lunch with Tom one day while Barbara was taking a lesson. He, who is 6 foot 5 inches and around 220 pounds and a formidable trencherman, watched in awe as I stowed away a meal that was easily double his. By way of dramatic demonstration, here is a typical day's diet for me the week before I went onto insulin:

Breakfast
> 2 figs
> 2 pieces of toast
> 1 boiled egg
> Coffee

Snack
> 1 glass milk
> 1 graham cracker

Lunch
> 1 small tomato
> 2 carrot sticks
> 1 ham sandwich
> 1 small apple
> Coffee

Dinner
> A few nuts and a bourbon and water
> 1 hamburger pattie
> ½ cup asparagus
> ½ cup beets
> 2 figs
> Coffee

Bedtime Snack
    1 glass milk
    ½ graham cracker

And here is what I consumed in one day at Badger Pass after twenty units of U-40 NPH insulin and with about five hours of skiing:

Breakfast
    ½ cup orange juice
    1½ pieces of toast
    ¾ bran muffin
    2 fried eggs
    3 strips bacon
    Small piece of fried mush
    Coffee

Snack
    1 cup Rice Krispies
    1 cup milk

Lunch
    1 generous tablespoon carrot with raisin salad
    1 generous tablespoon cottage cheese and orange salad
    Large serving of lettuce and tomato salad
    1 tablespoon crab and shrimp salad
    1 cup chicken chop suey and rice
    1 slice French bread
    ½ large banana
    Coffee

Snack (3:00 P.M.)
    1 apple
    1 cup milk

Snack (4:30 P.M.)
    ½ turkey and cheese sandwich

Tea (5:30 P.M.)
    ½ peanut butter cookie
    Tea with milk

Dinner
  A few nuts and a bourbon and water
  ⅛ avocado
  Large portion of lettuce and tomato salad
  ¼ hard-boiled egg
  1 stalk asparagus with crab and shrimp salad
  1 leg and 1 thigh of chicken Bourguignon with onions and
    mushrooms
  ¼ cup rice
  3½-ounce glass Burgundy
  ½ pear
  2 small slices of Swiss cheese
  ½ slice bread
  Coffee
  A sip of Barbara's cognac

Bedtime Snack
  ½ cup milk

Because my jaws were getting exhausted from all the chewing and eating and, more important, because I was, even with all that food, getting fairly regular before-dinner insulin reactions, I did drop my insulin dosage to fifteen units toward the end of the trip. Nevertheless I was still able to eat as heartily as the next person at the table, even when the next person was Tom.

By always skiing after a meal or a snack and by always carrying a store of foil-wrapped dates or little boxes of raisins for quick carbohydrates, I was able to avoid any insulin shocks on the slopes and even able to take both private hour-long ski lessons and two-hour-long classes. One day I took two two-hour class lessons, but I can't say I recommend that as a rational approach.

Barbara and I made several other short trips—some local one-day ones—to get in shape for our big excursion to France and Switzerland. There were no problems. Once when I took a private lesson I announced as a cautionary matter-of-course to my lean, bronzed, young-God-of-the-slopes ski instructor that I was a diabetic. He responded off-handedly that he had had diabetes since the age of nine. I was delighted and started trying to grill him about skiing diabetics and what extra precautions they should take. He didn't seem to want to discuss the subject and I later found out why. He'd lose his job if the head of the ski school ever found out, since the head wanted only "perfect specimens" both physiologically and urologically speaking. This was partially, I suppose, out of fear of workmen's compensation claims, but it probably also had something to do with the prevalent Dark Ages attitude about diabetes.

The trip to the Alps was a good deal more eventful, especially one day in Switzerland. We had gone from Grindelwald, where we were staying, up the mountain on the Wengen Alp Railway to Kleine Scheidegg. There we stopped to change trains for Wengen, where Barbara was going to the Molitor factory to order a pair of ski boots. We had our morning coffee and carbohydrate break overlooking the slopes that were beyond our poor powers to negotiate. I had tea with milk and two petits beurres, which was, I later figured out, about fifteen carbohydrates less than my normal snack and on a day when I was doing a lot of toting and slinging of skis, my feet constantly weighted by a ten-pound pair of boots.

Our train arrived. The trains in these ski-centered parts always have as the last car an open-air ski carrier complete with metal racks. We placed our skis in this, got on board, and the train hooted and headed down the mountain. There were not many others on board because this was the time of day when almost everyone was heading up the mountain to ski.

When the train pulled into the station at Wengen, we clumped out and discovered that, because of the way the train was parked, in order to get the skis, we'd have to run down the whole length of the train, cross in front of it, and run the whole length again to the ski-carrier car.

Since the train appeared to be pawing at the track anxious to leave, Barbara charged off. As she was going down the home stretch, thinking me right behind her, the train started up—it had not taken long to unload the few passengers. Barbara grabbed desperately at the skis, seeing some $250 worth of equipment about to chug off toward Murren, never to return. As she was reaching and wrenching and wondering why I wasn't doing the same, she glanced up through the network of stacked skis and saw the friendly neighborhood *Zuckerkrankerin* still standing on the platform on the other side of the train fumbling at a foil-wrapped date. Said *Zuckerkrankerin*, feeling eyes upon her, looked up and, I am told, shouted cheerfully, "On top of everything else, I'm fitting."

If the train hadn't slowed down momentarily for switching, Barbara would never have been able to get the second pair of skis off. But get them off she did, and as the train pulled away she began to lug both sets of skis and poles toward the platform. (Although she is only 5 feet 2½ inches and a 95-pound weakling, her strength is as the strength of ten when it comes to handling ski equipment.)

In my vagueness—the date had not yet taken hold—I realized I should be helping, so I wandered across the track toward where Barbara had been. On the way I decided that since I still wasn't functioning, another date was in order. I then proceded to laboriously unzip my parka pocket and inefficiently extract a date and begin anew the fumbling unwrapping process, only dimly aware that someone was shouting something in German— a language I don't understand a word of—into my ear. It was a railroad worker apparently informing me that I was standing in the middle of a track whereupon a train planned to run in the immediate future. Since I, all oblivious, continued to stand there and occupy myself with the date-unwrapping process, smiling vaguely as if an amiable asylum escapee, he finally, in desperation, flung me back against a parked train with one hand as he pulled the switch handle with the other. A train shot by so close that had I been Pinocchio, I would have lost the tip of my nose.

Of course, I wouldn't let almost getting run over by a train change my mind about skiing. In fact, I'm already planning next year's Alpine excursion. I'm totally hooked now. Why is it that as a diabetic I'm so wrapped up and sold on skiing? Partially for the same reasons a nondiabetic would be: because it is glorious, thrilling, exhilarating, magnificent, and every other superlative in the thesaurus.

For a diabetic, though, it has a couple of additional pluses. First, it thoroughly takes your mind off your disease. While you're involved in skiing, there is not a spare millimeter of space in your skull for thoughts of anything but what you're doing— or, more likely, trying to do. But even more important, as I read in an article on amputee veterans who are being encouraged to take up skiing on one leg. "Skiing has a marvelous therapeutic effect on the psyche as well as on the body. It makes any person with a physical handicap recapture the joy of living."

But if you elect to take up skiing, you do have to scrupulously observe the rules of the game, the same rules, incidentally, that *every* skier should observe:

1. Never ski alone.
2. Never ski unmarked or closed trails.
3. Never ski when the weather is such that you can't see what you're doing.
4. Never ski runs beyond your ability.
5. Always ski in control.
6. Take lessons.
7. Be in good physical condition.

It's also very important for a diabetic to dress warmly and comfortably and appropriately for the weather. Down-filled parkas are especially good since they combine warmth with light weight. When it comes to stretch pants, I, personally, make it a point to buy mine about a size larger than the ski shop personnel want me to. They like you to have them so tight that you can see if a dime is heads or tails through them. I don't believe a diabetic should be all that constricted about the waist, and, besides, I'm not stretching for a date with the ski instructor.

Boots, it goes without saying, should fit perfectly. It's imperative. Try on a hundred pairs—and pay a hundred dollars if you must—to get them right.

There should be no stinting on safety bindings, either. Most of the ski instructors that Barbara and I have queried recommend either Marker Rotomats or Look Nevadas as the best. But whatever kind you get, make sure that they're adjusted perfectly for you, otherwise the safety factor disappears.

Although skiing is my own thing now and I consider it the ideal sports activity, I'm not trying to convert every diabetic to it. The slopes are already getting more crowded than I would like them to be. The only reason I've described my skiing adventures in such detail is so that you'll believe a not-particularly-athletic forty-five-year-old woman diabetic skier and, once believing *that* unlikely creature, you should have no trouble at all believing yourself engaged in any kind of physical activitiy that attracts you. Anyone for Everest?

Chapter 9

HAVE DIABETES,
WILL TRAVEL

Look, up in the sky! It's a bird! It's a plane! It's Superdiabetic! No, I'm not referring to myself. Not so much modesty as honesty forces me to admit that as a diabetic traveler I have to take a second-class seat to one Mr. Wilfred Greenway. He disguises himself as the forty-eight-year-old mild-mannered U.S.A. Cargo Sales Manager for BOAC, but in reality he is Superdiabetic. He has been with BOAC since 1948 and has been a diabetic for the last six years. During these six years he has had only one week of sick leave and has traveled about 400,000 miles, including an around-the-world trip with absolutely no misadventures or mishaps of any kind.

Yes, comparing myself to that record, I don't feel I'm such a Wonderwoman. I've logged only about 34,000 miles in my two diabetic years. In contrast to Mr. Greenway, however, I've had lots of misadventures, and if you figure that a misadventure is as good as a mile, then I'm as qualified as he to speak on the subject of travel for diabetics.

My first major travel venture after diabetes—six months after—was a trip to Hawaii. I selected the Islands because they feel like foreign travel, exotics that they are, and yet they don't pose the hazards of language and unusual cuisine and customs. I was on pills then and free from insulin worries, but naturally I did have dietary ones. Since you never know exactly what will appear in the sections of those little plastic trays on airplanes, I feared it might all be high carbohydrate—a sugar-treated fruit cocktail, a starchy or saucy main dish, potatoes, succotash, pastry—and I would be able to eat almost nothing.

Barbara, on the job as always, said she thought she'd heard

that airlines serve special meals if they're notified ahead of time. She called the local office of the airline we were flying and found out that this was true and also that a diabetic meal was one of their standard deviations. She requested one for me.

During the flight I was consumed with curiosity to see what I would be having. I also very rapidly became consumed with hunger, because although everyone else was getting served, and served a nice luncheon of shrimp cocktail, meat, and non-carbohydratous vegetables that I could easily have handled, I kept being passed by. Barbara had alerted the stewardesses earlier that I was to get the diabetic meal. Now that I was getting nothing, however, she began to fret about my welfare. She offered me her lunch or any parts thereof I wanted, but I held off. I was intent on saving myself for my special meal.

Barbara held off, too, because she didn't want to eat with me staring cocker-spanielly at her food. Finally, when both her hot and cold foods had reached cabin temperature, she hove back to the galley to inquire of the whereabouts of my lunch. The stewardess said they were getting the regular meals out of the way first, but mine would be coming along presently. This struck both of us as odd, because you would think that it would be more logical to get the one odd meal out of the way before the one-hundred regular ones, rather than to get the one-hundred regular ones out of the way before the one odd one.

In our later research on airline food service, we found out that not only is it more logical, it's the way it's supposed to be handled. Continental Airlines was kind enough to send us the diabetic section from their stewardess training manual, and this comforting sentence is included. "*Note:* The hostess should offer the meal to a known diabetic first no matter where he is sitting."

This must be standard, because Barbara has a friend who is an ex-stewardess for Cunard Eagle, and she says they have the same policy. I think it would always be wise, though, to tell the stewardesses that you would be beholden to them if they would serve you your meal first. It's only fortunate that I wasn't on insulin at the time of this happening or I'd probably have yet another fit tale to tell.

When finally I got my special diabetic meal, it was something less than thrilling. I was, in fact, deprived of the shrimp cocktail that I had my mouth all set for from my close observation of Barbara's tray. In its stead I got a dull lettuce and tomato salad with only a lemon wedge to squirt for dressing. My meat was the same as that of the other passengers, but there were three (3) kinds of vegetables on my tray, all very tasty and enjoyable. For dessert I had canned fruit cocktail, which I loathe.

Since that time I have never again bothered to order a special diabetic meal in an airplane. With insulin I never have any trouble with what is served. Dessert in tourist class sometimes poses a problem, but the stewardesses have always been lovely about pinching me fruit and cheese from first class, where it's standard. By the way, although I've flown first class a couple of times since becoming a diabetic, I consider it a waste of money. A diabetic can't possibly make a noticeable empty space on the first-class groaning board, and all those bottomless wine bottles and fancy liqueurs are of small use to us.

Although I haven't ordered any special diabetic meals aloft since that first try, I may give it another chance. We've contacted all the major airlines to see what they serve diabetics (see Appendix E). Many of them have a special diabetic menu available, but to our surprise, we found that most prefer that you specify exactly what your meal should include so that they can send aboard a tray tailored to your individual requirements. Barbara is urging me next time to order beluga caviar, Belgian endive salad, pheasant under glass, *fond d'artichauts* filled with Strasbourg *pâte de foie gras truffé*, white asparagus, and for dessert wild strawberries. This is one time I wouldn't mind playing guinea pig for one of her diabetic experiments.

Whatever the meal being served in whatever class I'm flying, though, there is one safety measure I always take. I have what I call my carbohydrate arsenal tucked away in the inner zipper compartment of my purse along with the other *sine qua non*, my makeup. This carbohydrate arsenal is composed of individually foil-wrapped dates, a box of raisins, little cellophane packs of crackers, and—for the ultimate need—miniature bars of Swiss chocolate, which I prefer to sugar cubes. Why not make the treatment a treat that you wouldn't otherwise have? I keep all of this anti-shock material ready for action in case something goes wrong with the meal service, an occurrence which is not as unlikely as you might think.

On my second diabetic flight to Hawaii, the first-class oven was suffering some ailment that made it cook only half as fast as normally. The meal was as a consequence delayed, and I had to dip into my purse for emergency rations. The oven could have been totally conked out, in which case I would simply have eaten my way through my total carbohydrate arsenal. I've heard of even more hazardous situations. On a charter flight from Los Angeles to London that a friend of mine took, when the stewardesses started to serve dinner, they discovered that all the food was spoiled and totally inedible. The unfortunate passengers spent eleven hours aloft without a morsel.

Another way to cope with in-flight eating problems is suggested by Peter R. Richards, Medical Officer for BEA and BOAC:

> Where there is any doubt regarding the treatment of diabetes we advise passengers to withhold their insulin or oral hypo-glycaemic drugs. The dangers of a hypoglycaemic attack are greater than hyperglycaemia as they can come on suddenly and unexpectedly if food is not taken. Hyperglycaemia takes much longer to develop and in the early stages is not so dangerous to the patient. So if there is any doubt about whether a meal can be obtained or how long it will be until the next meal is available, we advise passengers to withhold treatment.

Since Dr. Richards is privileged to attach to his name the formidable list of initials, M.B., D.P.H., D.I.H., D.T.M. & H., D.Obst. R.C.O.G., I think we can take his advice with all faith.

Along with the meal problem—and in a sense a part of it—is the problem of jet lag or, as it's technically called, arrhythmia. This is what happens to you when you fly fast and far and suddenly find yourself in a new and strange time zone. The clock tells you it's one time, your body tells you it's another, and your mind is too tired and confused to make itself up. What is a diabetic to do? As always there are several choices.

Just figuring it out for myself, this is what I did when Barbara and I went on our latest European trip. We took a flight for New York that left Los Angeles at 5:00 P.M. We planned to stay in New York a couple of nights both because we had some business to attend to and because I wanted to adjust to time zone changes more gradually. I had a snack before boarding the plane so I wouldn't get nervous when the inevitable meal-serving delay aloft inevitably took place. My dinner on the plane was later than I usually eat. This I considered all to the good, because it helped adjust me to the three-hour-later New York time zone and made it unnecessary for me to have my usual bedtime milk and graham crackers. By the time we got to our hotel (the Algonquin, where we always stay because it makes us feel like Dorothy Parker), it was 2:00 A.M. New York time and 11:00 P.M. stomach time.

The next morning we got up at 8:30 by the New York clock, and I took my insulin injection at 9:00 (6:00 A.M. Los Angeles time, just a half-hour earlier than I usually take it). The rest of that day I ate on a slightly modified New York time schedule: breakfast around 10:00, lunch at 1:30 or 2:00, dinner at 9:00. The following day I normalized the eating hours for breakfast and lunch and then, snack-fortified as usual, I boarded the Swissair plane for Zurich at 5:45 P.M. and proceeded to abnormalize my eating hours all over again.

Dinner was at about 7:00 P.M., and at midnight they served a continental breakfast. This I used as a late, late bedtime snack and booster, because not only was I to have no sleep that night, but I knew that debarking from the plane at 1:00 A.M. and luggage-gathering (including skis and boots) would use up a bunch of blood sugar. The breakfast was composed of juice, fruit, cheese, rolls, and coffee. I had a sip of orange juice and a roll smeared with one of the little Gruyère packages. Another package of Gruyère and an apple I pocketed for later use.

It was 8:00 A.M. in Zurich and 2:00 A.M. in my personal never-never land when we loaded our waiting rental Volkswagen and headed out cross-country toward Geneva and our ultimate destination, Megève, France. About an hour and a half out of Zurich, I extracted a disposable syringe from my purse, blearily filled it with insulin, and gave myself my fix in my left thigh as we bounced along the Swiss Hartstrasse. This was at 9:30 A.M. Swiss time and 3:30 A.M. body time, meaning that I had moved my regular injection time up about three hours. At 10:00 A.M. we stopped at a small hotel for a breakfast of *oeufs sur le plat* (fried eggs and ham in a small, flat casserole). I ate two chunks of bread along with this, and back in the car I consumed the purloined Swissair apple.

At about 2:00 P.M. (8:00 A.M. body time), having passed through Bern, Lausanne, Geneva, and across the border into France, we stopped for lunch at Annemasse and I put away a complete meal of smoked salmon, roast chicken, green beans, French-fried potatoes, cheese, and fruit.

We pressed on and reached Megève at about 3:00 P.M. (9:00 A.M. old time). We settled into our little garret room at Hotel L'Hermitage, fell onto our beds, and slept until 8:00 P.M. (2:00 P.M. old time). Then we mustered ourselves up to eat dinner, returned to the room, took a sleeping pill prescribed by my doctor, toppled over again, and slept until 7:00 A.M. the following morning. To my amazement, I awoke fresh, totally adjusted to the new time zone and ready for skiing. During this entire ordeal I had not spilled, nor had I had any twinges of hypoglycemia.

Since I had worked out my own arhythmia-avoidance schedule, I was pleased to have it for the most part confirmed by BEA and BOAC's multi-initialed Dr. Richards, who advises:

When a diabetic passenger travels through several time zones he should not attempt to alter his diabetic regime until he has reached his destination. Although the time is changing outside the aircraft as it flies between New York and London, time in the passenger's body remains at takeoff time and only alters very slowly after his arrival. We advise that he should modify his regime by not more than two hours a day until he is taking his insulin or other treatment at the new time appropriate to his place of destination (in other words, continue your insulin injections at takeoff time, altering it two hours a day, either backwards or forwards, until your usual regime is resumed). If the patient changes his time too suddenly, he is likely to get hypoglycaemic or hyperglycaemic attacks.

Superdiabetic Greenway, though, handles his eastward journeys in a slightly different way:

> I travel between New York and London quite frequently, and I take the evening flights. Although an evening meal is served on board and a breakfast before arrival—all in the space of some six hours, my normal habit is to have my dinner at my accustomed time, and I forego my meal on the aircraft. In view of the five-hour time difference I make lunch in UK my first meal preceded by my insulin shot and then have my three meals with lunch, dinner, and late snack around midnight. I then begin the following day with breakfast, and I am adjusted. I have traveled from New York to Scotland to attend a luncheon with no ill effect, but one must be conditioned to do it successfully.

To show you how flexible you can be in adjusting to a new time zone, a young college student named Tom Gess, writing in *The Diabetic* of his year of study abroad in Aix-en-Provence, France, says:

> I think I should say something about the first couple of days after your arrival. Remember there will be a time change of eight or nine hours, and you will not be able to maintain as good control as you might like to in those first one or two days, but this is of minor consequence. Just mind the clock. If it says 8 in the morning it is 8 in the morning where you are. It is not *really* midnight back home in the States as your mind will allow you to think. Just think of it as daylight savings time multiplied several times, and you'll have no problems!!!

Exclamation points his, but I feel like adding a few of my own. Clearly, he, too, has Superdiabetic tendencies. In fact, in his article he mentions taking an insulin injection in Pisa in Clark Kent's favorite undressing room, a phone booth.

If you are on insulin or the pills and want to travel abroad, I strongly urge, as does Mr. Greenway, that you take with you "sufficient supplies for a trip—add a few days for safety—and then make sure they travel with you and are not packed away in baggage." (Honest airline man there, to admit that you don't always arrive bag and baggage. Also, insulin should never be left in your luggage when you fly because the luggage is frequently stored in an unpressurized part of the aircraft where the insulin might freeze—and freezing is the one thing that totally destroys its effectiveness.) On the sufficient-supplies score, there really is no reason for you to have to cope with foreign pharmacies unless you're living overseas for an extended period. For emergencies, though, which have a way of happening when you travel, we've included in the Appendix the brand names of the various pills and insulins sold abroad that would correspond to your American dosage. It might be wise to carry a photocopy of this so that, if you need a refill, you could just point and get what you wanted with minimum strain all around.

Incidentally, if you are on U-80 insulin and you're visiting France, be particularly careful to take along an adequate supply. As Tom Gess mentions in his article,

> France has only 40-unit insulin. For some reason known only to the French, 80-unit is simply not manufactured. This is what the pharmacist and my doctor told me in Aix-en-Provence. I did use the 40-unit insulin for a while, but I had to double the dosage and thus the quantity was too uncomfortable to inject.

On the subject of insulin I have a few additional caveats, or rather *non*-caveats. When I made my first extended European trip as an insulin-taker (the one to France and Switzerland), I handled my little vials as gingerly and nervously as a first-time mother would treat a premature infant. From the directions inside the insulin-bottle box, and from reading books on diabetes, I had picked up the idea that insulin must always be kept cool, preferably under refrigeration. There were even descriptions of how to carry it around in a wide-mouthed thermos bottle filled with ice cubes. The books and pamphlets never made it clear what would happen if you didn't keep your insulin cool, but the implication, for me, was that it would be like injecting your-self with rattlesnake venom. When I started traveling with in-sulin, then, in airplanes I would hand my supply to the stew-ardess and ask her to slip it into the icebox, and then all through the flight I'd be afraid I'd forget and leave it there. In hotels, I would send it to the kitchen and have it placed in the refrigera-tor. I remember particularly well our stay at the Algonquin. When the bellboy took us to our room, it was very stuffy and I knew my precious insulin would surely expire in such an atmosphere, but I thought it might survive in the night air on the window ledge. I asked the bellboy if he could open a window.

"I want to put my insulin outside to keep it cool," I told him.

"Your insulin? Oh, *that* has to be refrigerated," he said with firm authority. "You can call down in the morning and someone will bring it right up."

The next morning, I rang the desk and asked for my insulin. It arrived a half-hour later than I wanted to take it. And it was a matter of enter bellboy with insulin, exit bellboy with a fifty-cent tip and a little later, enter bellboy (different bellboy), exit bellboy and insulin and fifty-cent tip. I decided I was a victim of the insulin shell game, the greatest New York racket since selling the Brook-lyn Bridge went out of style.

In the hotels in the French and Swiss Alps I was able to keep my insulin in the room, since the climate was cooler, but I had to put it out on the balcony to cool and bring it in to keep it from freezing so often that it was as if it were a pet I was trying to housebreak. Barbara began to complain that I was worthless as a travel compan-ion because I wouldn't ever "chat amiably of current issues" with her. My mind was occupied exclusively with thoughts of insulin— whether to put it outside or bring it inside. She would huffily re-treat into a book, grousing that obviously my insulin was the only company I needed.

When I was home again and discussing the trip with my doc-tor, my one big complaint about travel was the difficulty of keeping my insulin cool, and I told him of the New York insulin extortion racket.

I have seldom seen him so amused. "Insulin's not *that* delicate," he assured me. "Why, I carry it around in my medical bag for weeks at a time and nothing ever happens to it. You just have to be careful not to let it sit and bake in a hot car or in the direct sun."

"But what if it *did* get too warm and I wasn't aware of it?"

"It would just lose its effectiveness slightly. It certainly wouldn't kill you," he said, apparently reading my mind. "The worst that would happen would be that you might spill a little."

When Barbara went to my doctor for her annual checkup a few weeks later, he was still chuckling over my having to pay a $1.00 daily ransom for my insulin in New York.

Later, in Tom Gess's article, I read his typically free-wheeling comment:

> I had a ten-month supply of NPH and regular insulin which lasted perfectly the whole time under room temperature, both in my room at school and on the road traveling. Insulin is really quite a hardy substance, and can be stored just about anywhere with little fear of deterioration.

Naturally, on a trip to a foreign country, you'll want to also take along any other medications you normally use or occasionally use or even possibly *might* use. Mr. Greenway advises: "I do think it is a good idea for overseas travellers to take medicine for upset stomachs and intestinal problems. I always feel this is my 'Achilles heel' when travelling so I make every effort to keep my inner workings in good order."

I've fortunately never been plagued with air sickness, but for those who are—or think they might be—here's a tip from the British Diabetic Association: "Anti-sickness drugs are often helpful and are harmless to diabetics; the important point to remember is to take them at once and not to wait until sickness is felt, especially if the traveller is apprehensive."

Another health insurance policy for the diabetic going abroad is joining Intermedic (777 Third Avenue, New York, N.Y. 10017) on the theory that if you have it you won't need it. It only costs $5.00 for an individual or $9.00 for a family, and for that you get a list of over 355 competent physicians in 174 cities throughout the world who guarantee to treat you for $8.00 for the first office visit. And they all speak English. (See Appendix D.)

And speaking of English, if that's the only language you *do* speak, there is still no need to fear traveling as a diabetic. Enough Americans and British have been almost everywhere in the world before you to lay the linguistic groundwork, and if you hit only the major cities of the most popular tourist countries, you'll probably have more trouble trying to find someone who *doesn't* speak English than someone who does.

I do think, however, that for your own peace of mind and pancreas it would behoove you to master a few phrases appropriate to the diabetic (see Appendix F) so that you can at least ask for orange juice in an emergency or ascertain whether or not, for example, a fruit compote contains sugar.

Your travel companion may also be willing to participate in the linguistic experience. Barbara does this even more than I consider necessary. When we left New York for Zurich, I knew what I was in for for the rest of the trip when the young Swiss steward sat in the seat next to her for the takeoff and she turned to him, smiled warmly, and jerking her thumb in my direction, announced with pride, *"Zuckerkrank ist."*

Another wise thing to do is to carry a diabetic identification card in the language of the country. For your convenience, in Appendix G you'll find the usual message in thirteen languages. These can be clipped and slipped into your wallet or purse.

If you should already know something of the language of the land you're planning to visit, an excellent way to brush up on it is to write to the diabetes association of that country for materials. In that way you get the advantage of learning more about both the language and diabetes. Likewise, it's good to carry with you the addresses of the diabetic associations of the countries you're visiting (see Appendix E), and in case you need help or advice, contact them and they'll assist you.

Turning now to food overseas, it's not as much of a problem as you might imagine. You can find American/British-style breakfasts in most large international hotels, and as the experienced Mr. Greenway says, "I recommend having a breakfast of eggs, cereal, and fruit which are usually available everywhere, so that the body can assimilate something with which it is familiar."

If you're planning to do a little more hinterland wandering, the way Tom Gess did, then you may have to make a few early-morning adjustments, for as he says:

> In most European countries, as some of you may already know, breakfast is meager, consisting mainly of a roll and coffee. This is what you'll get in countries on the continent like Spain, France, or Italy. . . . Now this did pose somewhat of a problem in the beginning. If I ate a so-called continental breakfast at 8:00 (to get a nice early start) and went sight-seeing right afterwards, by 10:00 with all the walking, the inevitable result was insulin reaction. Try and supplement your breakfasts by ordering a little more if this is possible. I often took two breakfasts. Keep some fruit or some form of carbohydrate in your room. Actually you should do this anyway in order to be prepared for any situations that might arise. It is important then to always eat a little more than you normally would in the morning or arrange with your doctor to adjust your dosage before leaving. You must account for these small, rather unbalanced European breakfasts, or you will be in trouble.

As for those breakfast supplements, on my last trip I found them to be exorbitant. My breakfast boiled egg, for example, added $.65 to the cost of the meal. Drinking fruit juice off the hotel menu would have cost like champagne, so I bought small cans at the grocery store, where they weren't exactly cheap, either ($.30 for the six-ounce cans which cost around $.15 in this country), and cooled them in the Alpine night air out on the balcony.

For the other meals, as Mr. Greenway says, "one must be prepared for all different types of food for lunches and suppers, particularly in Asian countries where Chinese-type meals are everywhere." It's something like my San Francisco eating venture except easier because you'll always be eating in restaurants of the same nationality and in a few days you'll know pretty well how to handle the menu. There are a number of menu-deciphering books available to help you with this. One of the most readily obtainable is the one published by Pan Am.

As for dining on the Continent, the British Diabetic Association makes these observations in their booklet "Holidays":

> In *Switzerland* you will certainly find every comfort; here hoteliers are well trained and out to please their clients. *Austria* is a much simpler country, and whereas everything will be very clean and attractive, the food may be of a lower standard than in Switzerland. However, there will still be no difficulty in getting adequate amounts of protein. Sometimes green vegetables are not very plentiful, and this is an occasion where you might have a word with the proprietor, who will generally do his best for you. Both in *Holland* and *Norway* meals are extremely generous and rich in protein. In these two countries protein is also served with breakfast. In *Italy* the favourite dish is pasta. Two ounces of cooked spaghetti, macaroni or pasta contain 15 grams of carbohydrate. Usually grated cheese and tomato are served with pasta and you can be generous, therefore, with the trimmings. *France* is particularly easy for the diabetic and salads are always available. . . . Cheese and fresh fruit and ices are served for the sweet course. Remember that a small scoop of ice cream contains approximately 10 grams of carbohydrate. Ice cream is one of the few sweet dishes served on the Continent, and it can be very good, indeed, with the most delicious flavourings. In Italy, where ice-cream shops and barrows are everywhere, a portion can make a very useful mid-morning buffer or tea-time break.

Spain can cause a diabetic problems, not because of the food, which, as Tom Gess says, is "substantial and quite varied," but because of the late dining hours. The only thing for a diabetic to do here is nudge his schedule forward as the British Diabetic Association suggests.

If, in Spain, the country of late meals according to our standards, you find the midday meal is served at 2 P.M., take your breakfast correspondingly later and make your injection fit in with this. If you are not a stay-a-bed and like to get up at 7 A.M., order an early morning cup of tea to brace you up for the 9 o'clock or later breakfast.

Mr. Greenway, who does a good deal of his traveling in the Orient, says that he avoids fresh vegetables "such as lettuce and salads, and also fruit." (This doesn't apply to Europe. When I was in France and Switzerland I ate all of these commodities constantly and to no ill effect.) I do agree with Mr. Greenway in the case of certain countries, though—Mexico especially springs to mind, and some of the less modernized nations of the East. In Japan, however, I wouldn't hesitate to eat salads and fresh fruits and vegetables in the international hotels. When I traveled there as an undiscovered diabetic, I ate everything served (except for occasional raw octopus tentacles), and with impunity. I imagine that what Mr. Greenway is trying to avoid with his banned items is the same thing nondiabetics are trying to avoid, namely the classic intestinal malady of tourism, which is admittedly far more serious for a diabetic, confusing the food-absorption issue as it does.

One of the best features I find about foreign travel—especially European travel—for the insulin-taking diabetic is that snacking is a way of life. You'd think every member of the population was a diabetic on insulin from the way they're always popping into a cafe for a leisurely bite or sip. Then, too, the English schedule of eating—with the large breakfast and the "elevenses" morning break and the afternoon tea which takes place at the time when my particular kind of insulin is likely to go on a rampage—I consider ideal.

All things considered, if I were you, I certainly wouldn't hesitate to take a trip anywhere, any time. After all, I'm me and I don't hesitate. It's very possible that when you launch yourself on your first venture, you may find that under your drip-dry shirt or print dress there shines a big red "S" and you've got possibilities, red-hot possibilities, you don't even know you've got, to become Superdiabetic yourself. Up, up, and away!

Chapter 10

LA DIABÉTIQUE IMAGINAIRE

And now for the flip side of the diabetic record. The voice of the nondiabetic half here takes up the refrain in order to give you diabetics the giftie of seeing yoursels as ithers see you, and to provide aid and comfort to close friends and relatives of diabetics in their problems with the care and feeding of these fascinating and unpredictable creatures.

During the period of wrestling with June's diabetes and writing this book, I've begun to feel like the George Plimpton of the diabetes game—a kind of paper guinea pig. I've eaten the diabetic diet, followed the regular diabetic exercise program, joined diabetes associations, read everything I could on the subject, jabbed myself with the needle, passed for a diabetic at the local diabetes fair, and I even went for my annual checkup to June's doctor.

In fact, the only two diabetic plays I haven't run are taking the pills and injecting myself with insulin. But then, even Plimpton didn't get into the real league action with the Detroit Lions. Besides, I know better than to play games with those blood-sugar-droppers, after reading about the local Los Angeles insulin killer, a former lab technician who injected several nondiabetic family members with insulin to bring about their sudden, untimely, and mysterious demise.

At any rate, after a year and a half of playing the role of *La Diabétique Imaginaire*, both at home and on the road, I find —and here I'd best lower my voice so she can't hear—that June's diabetes is one of the most useful things that has ever happened to me. No one could be more surprised than I that it has turned out this way. When June's diabetes was first diagnosed, it

101

appeared to be an ill wind that couldn't possibly blow anyone good, least of all me. Since we had always had as two of our primary free-lance writing targets foreign travel and gourmet dining, when she came home from the doctor's office that March 17 clutching her 1,800-calorie diet and her box of Orinase and her little paperback book of restrictions, it was as if she had been handed a death sentence for the good life. And since collaboration demands a pretty close relationship, I felt that, in the manner of the servants of the Egyptian pharaohs, I was going to be buried alive right along with her.

Not so. In fact, just the opposite. Not only am I still living, I'm flourishing on the diabetic way of life. This would-be funeral lily has picked up a modicum of gilt by diabetic association.

Thanks to keeping more regular hours, gone are the smudgy thumb prints I used to frequently wear under my eyes, and clearer are the eyes above where they used to appear.

I have developed a passionate love and devotion—almost a fetish—for fresh fruits and vegetables. And now that I have become intimately familiar with food values, I have an instinctive abhorrence for those abominations that any rational human *should* have an instinctive abhorrence for, such as grease-soaked carbohydrates. Since it's true to a certain extent that you are what you eat, I'm now somewhat closer to being a crunchy apple than a soggy fried potato.

My exercise program, too, has been greatly improved, though in a slightly different way from my sleeping and eating habits. No one has ever had to use a cattle prod to get me into action around swimming pools, tennis courts, bowling alleys, horse stables, or ski slopes. But to me sports are as much for the companionship as for the exercise itself. In her pre-diabetic days—or really I guess they were her *undiscovered* diabetic days —June had neither the stamina nor the inclination to spend much time in physical activities. Now, however, I always have in her a ready, willing, and increasingly able sports playmate.

Besides looking and feeling better on the diabetic regime, I actually *am* better. When I used to eat on a highly irregular schedule, sometimes going so far as to skip a couple of meals in a row, I would become quite disagreeable, even, some considered, impossible to be around. Nondiabetics can have low blood sugar, too, and while they don't pass out from it, it does serve to radically unsweeten their dispositions. Now that I eat three square and well-rounded meals a day, what I called my "artistic personality" (others were wont to refer to it as a vile temper) has diminished considerably.

Yes, all in all, we close friends and relatives of diabetics are, in a sense, fortunate. We get all of the advantage of diabetes with none of its drawbacks. If we share a diabetic's meals and living habits and exercise schedule, our own health is bound to improve. For, aside from the insulin or tolbutamide or tolazimide, it's not just a bromide to say that the diabetic way of life is nothing more than the intelligent and healthful way of life, the kind everyone ought to be following, but few, without some special goading, do. Not only that, but should our own systems have latent leanings toward diabetes—as well they might since it's getting so prevalent that the prediction is that sometime in the Buck Rogers future *everybody* will have diabetes—following the diabetic regime could very likely keep any latent leanings from toppling over into overt diabetes. Yes, having a diabetic friend or relative is the best health insurance policy you can get, and he's paying the premiums for you. You should show your appreciation. How? There are a number of ways.

1. Help the diabetic to grin and bear it.

I've heard it said that to cope successfully with life you should learn to take the light things seriously and the serious things lightly. This applies very well to diabetes. The diabetic who develops not only a positive attitude, but even a sense of humor about his condition has a better perspective on himself and on his malady. Naturally, having diabetes is not in itself a hilarious joke, but neither is it the greatest of world tragedies. Funny things do happen to a diabetic because he is a diabetic, and these incidents can be enjoyed for their inherent amusement value.

In this respect, I'm grateful for June's sublime sense of the ridiculous. Not every diabetic would go along with referring to "popping pills" or "taking a fix," and maybe even fewer would enjoy having their hypoglycemic attacks referred to as "fitting." But you can work out your own routines and diabetic "in" jokes. If you are close to a diabetic, you will know what kind of remarks he would consider amusing rather than abusing. But however you manage it, it's your responsibility to put the leavening into his sugar-free loaf.

2. Learn as many food values as you can.

A diabetic, in order to operate effectively in gourmet realms or even just to be a bit free-wheeling in his selection of meals, has to be a walking table of food logarithms. It's not easy. If you can help out by storing some of the facts in your own memory bank, the diabetic's eating range will be that much broader, and you can plan the meals he eats with you safely, but adventuresomely. If you're the mother or wife of a diabetic, I realize that this advice is superfluous. You undoubtedly already know more of the food values than the diabetic in your life can ever hope to.

If you're the friend of a diabetic and you have him over to a dinner party, don't deprive the other guests of a rich dessert. Let them go ahead and blub up and rot their teeth, if they like. Just provide some fresh fruit for the diabetic. Cutting out all sweets because a diabetic is in attendance is as bad as cutting out all liquor because there's one alcoholic in the house. It only makes him uncomfortable because he feels he's spoiling everyone else's fun.

3. In restaurants order a backup meal.

Sometimes when we're eating out, June casts her eye over a menu and manages to hook it on the dish most likely to make her spill. I particularly remember her fatal attraction to a Middle Eastern lamb shank with prune sauce, kumquats, and almonds. In a case like this, rather than hooting with derision or flailing her with solid logic, I simply order for myself something I'm certain will be all right, something I know she'd probably like, such as *blanquette de veau*. Then when the dishes arrive and the first sweet, rich forkful illumines her face with despair, I can ask if she'd like to trade, and I'll credit her some good sense, she usually does.

And while we're discussing dining out with diabetics, here's something a close friend or relative has to be on guard against for his *own* good: eating and drinking for two. If you become a handy, dandy automatic carbohydrate and calorie disposal service, draining off the dregs of cocktails and chomping down a diabetic's mostly leftover French fries or untouched desserts, you're going to become a sallow, paunchy Jack Spratt's wife while your diabetic waxes lean and rosy. The one exception I make to this is, when we're in France, I always help June out by finishing off the last of any vintage wines. After all, one must make some sacrifices.

4. Make all special requests for diabetic needs.

You can be the one to ask for anything out of the ordinary that a diabetic requires. I've noticed that June hesitates to call attention to herself by asking the stewardess on an airplane to bring her her meal first or fetch her some fresh fruit or, in the days when we foolishly thought it necessary, put her insulin in the ice-cube bin. Because she hates to do it, she's particularly inept at it.

On the way home from our most recent trip to Hawaii, for instance, we boarded the plane at 12:30 P.M. in Honolulu. Our cabin staff was one of those international sets that airlines take such pride in. We had as stewardesses (they announced in conjunction with the ditching and oxygen-breathing instructions) a Japanese girl, a Finnish girl, a German—and a Texan.

We expected lunch to be served very shortly after takeoff. In fact, that was why we had selected that particular hour to fly. But as 1:00, 1:15, and 1:30 marched by, there was no sign of food, and June began writhing in her seat complaining of gnawings of hunger and varied subtle harbingers of low blood sugar. I volunteered to trot back and ask that she be served first (we were seated in midfuselage), but since she was going to the restroom, anyway, she said she would be a big girl and accost the galley-operating stewardess herself.

Back she came, tone *funeste*-ing with me, "She won't do it."

"What?" I said in disbelief. "You can't be serious. What did she say?"

Apparently the words of the stewardess had been burned on June's soul, because she was able to repeat their exchange verbatim:

"I said, 'I'm on insulin. May I be served dinner first?' And the stewardess said, 'Absolutely not, madame. It's not dinner; it's lunch. And it's not even ready yet. The trays are frozen and it takes a long time to heat them. But they'll be ready in about twenty minutes.'"

"Didn't you tell her you're a diabetic?" I asked.

"Yes, I said very clearly, 'I'm on insulin.'"

I looked at her witheringly. "Well, *that* explains it. You probably got one of the foreign stewardesses and she had no idea what you were talking about. 'I'm on insulin!' What a weird way to put it. She must have thought insulin was some kind of group tour of the Islands and you were just trying to con them into special treatment for no good reason."

Just about that time the Finnish stewardess came by to collect the drink glasses. As she leaned over our row of seats, despite June's tugging at my sleeve and whispering, "No, no, it'll only be twenty minutes more. Don't make a scene," I fastened my granite eye on the stewardess and enunciated, "My friend here is a *di-a-bet-ic*. Could she be served her lunch first, as soon as it is ready?"

"Of course," she said crisply.

At 2:15 June was finally served, and to show that it did make a difference, I didn't get my meal until 2:45, when June was already finished and sitting securely and comfortably with the blood sugar singing in her veins.

Later I got June to ask the girl who had refused her request (she was the German) why. Just as I thought, she told her apologetically, "But you didn't *say* you were a diabetic. I didn't know that was why you wanted to eat first."

I pointed out to June, using my best ex-second-grade–teacher tones, that a person is not told unless he understands what you're saying.

In a restaurant, too, June hates to "make a scene." She will sit miserably picking at a plate containing succotash and mashed potatoes before she will ask for a substitution. When business conferences are being arranged, she doesn't like to insist on scheduling them so as to avoid periods of low blood sugar. I, on the other hand, can be quite adamant, even high-handed in these matters. It's always much easier to demand special treatment for others than for yourself. You are, as a matter of fact, considered altruistic and noble when you do so, both by the people from whom you extract the service and your diabetic friend—not to mention by yourself.

In conjunction with this, if you're traveling with a diabetic in a foreign country, it's important for you as well as the diabetic to learn the appropriate phrases to get diabetic needs met (see Appendix F). Indeed, if there's ever a true, flapping emergency, you'll be the only one fully conscious and capable of using them.

Incidentally, of all the special things I've ever asked for for June, and I've asked for a good number of them, I've only been denied one. People are always extremely considerate and helpful and sympathetic. I remember in a tea shop in Chamonix when I was grilling the proprietress on the amount of sugar in the various pastries and I explained why, she gasped and groaned and gazed over toward June with such pity and compassion that I thought she was going to soggy up the sponge cake with her tears. I suppose in a country as food-oriented as France anything that restricts your diet at all is considered a tragedy as profound and moving as *Phèdre*.

5. Learn how to recognize the symptoms of hypoglycemia and what to do about them.

According to the books, hypoglycemia—or insulin shock— is usually indicated by weakness or trembling, paleness, and sweating, etc. From my observations of June, however, I've decided that the reactions of each individual vary tremendously; hypoglycemia is a very personal thing. In June's case, she sometimes shows an on-coming fit by getting extremely irritable and hostile. I recall that once just before lunch another librarian and June and I were shoving around some library furniture and discussing its rearrangement, a fairly unemotional subject, you must admit. Yet to every suggestion the other librarian and I made on the placement of the furniture June reacted— *over*-reacted—with rude and offensive negativism, pronouncing such edicts as "That's an idiotic idea if I ever heard one" and "I don't know why I even bothered to ask you two. You obviously don't know anything about how the reference desk is supposed to function." I fully felt like pouncing on her and pressing my thumbs to her windpipe. Then suddenly, through my own mounting miasma of wrath, it occurred to me that June was not behaving at all normally and that her insolence was probably spelled i-n-s-u-l-i-n; so I pushed her into her office and made eat the fruit out of her lunch. In a few minutes she was her old, if not agreeable, at least diplomatic self.

A further complication with June's hypoglycemia is that she grows stubborn about the very subject that she needs to be most malleable about—eating. Often my mild suggestion that she eat something is met with a flat, surly refusal. When that happens, I know I'd better get some carbohydrate down her gullet fast and by any method possible, including Strasbourg goose force-feeding.

Then, again, sometimes her oncoming attacks are heralded with vagueness, a kind of wandering around lightly bumping into things and/or picking up objects and putting them down somewhere else for no apparent reason.

Still another earlier and milder sign, one that has taken me a good while to be able to recognize, is a gradual subtle change in her appearance. Her eyes become unnaturally and unhealthily bright and her face grows thinner, sharper; it kind of sinks into itself. It's hard to explain, but it's a total feeling I get of all not being quite right with her.

But you never really know every possible insulin-shock symptom a diabetic can have, because the rascals are always coming up with new ones. After June's first eventful six months as a needle jockey, I thought I'd seen everything she had to offer in the fitting line. But no, we were playing golf one day and as we were ready to tee off at the sixteenth hole, she suddenly acquired a "tingling derriere"—felt as if it were asleep, she said. We had no idea what was wrong, but just to be on the safe side, we shot her some fast carbohydrate. Sure enough it cleared it up.

What to do when you see one of these fits coming on or actually *on?* If you're alert and catch them before they're too bad, just any old carbohydrate drink or snack will do. If they're well under way and you want fast recovery, a sweet liquid is in order: fruit juice or a soft drink. I tend to go for the fruit juice. The diabetic might as well get a few vitamins along with the sugar pop. Besides, these days, because of the no-calorie vogue, you can't always be sure you're getting something that will do the diabetic any good. Tom's friend Jim had a memorable experience on this score. He and a friend were out for a drive when he began to feel odd and hungry. He knew he should have something to eat so he asked the friend to stop at a hamburger stand. He says now he should have realized he was in an extra-hazardous state because he remembers staggering as he got out of the car. But reason was already beginning to dissolve in insulin. He ate a hamburger, but even he realized that wasn't enough, so he ordered a soft drink and got the sugar-free version. He took the bottle with him and he stumbled back to the car. As they drove, Jim kept swigging at the carbohydrate-less drink and feeling curiouser and curiouser until he finally toppled forward unconscious and his friend had to rush him to an emergency hospital for revival.

One thing I've learned about bringing up blood sugar is not to tell the beginning-to-fit diabetic to "go eat or drink something" or ask him "what would you like?" The power of decision is the first faculty to go. I've seen June staring vaguely into the refrigerator or softly bouncing off the kitchen counters and walls, as she wanders and wonders what she should have to counteract the insulin that is taking charge. No more than you would ask a drunk what he would like to sober up on would you ask an insulin-shocking diabetic his taste in the matter. Just say, "Go eat a banana," or "Go drink some of that guava nectar in the refrigerator." Better still, hand whatever carbohydrate you're pushing to the diabetic and say, "Here, take this," and stand there until he does.

Finally, something I learned the hard way on the ski slopes in France, *always* carry sugar or hard candy whenever you go out anywhere with a diabetic, especially if you're doing exercise.

It happened one day in Megève. After all our loading and unloading of skis, ticket-buying, riding up on the *téléphérique*, etc., it was almost noon, the hour at which one feeds the *Zuckerkrankerin* or else gets fitted upon. We had eaten at the restaurant at the *téléphérique* terminal the day before; so we thought we'd try the other one. (There were really three others up there, but we didn't know that at the time.) The one we were after, the Ideal-Sport, was, it said on the sign, a fifteen-minute walk from where we were.

I doubtfully asked June if she thought she could make it. She even more doubtfully said she thought she could, as she unwrapped a foil-covered date and chomped it down for a quick carbohydrate pop. The wind was screeching through the trees and it was suddenly cloudy. There was hardly anyone around; there hardly ever was then, since it was so late in the season. Thinking we couldn't go to the restaurant on foot, because there were signs all around saying it was strictly *défendu* to walk on the *piste*, we, with the usual great effort, strapped on our skis and started slogging up the narrow trail. And up it was. *Very* up.

After what seemed like a ten-minute climb we came to an open area where the *piste* crossed the trail, and there was a sign and arrow indicating where the *foot* path continued to the restaurant. We cleverly surmised from this that it was permissible to walk on the trail; so off went the skis at more great effort. We hoisted them to our shoulders and, using our poles like walking sticks, continued the uphill march. It was difficult and exhausting, even for me. I began to worry about June's carbohydrates. One mere date could hardly be expected to carry off a weighted mountain climb like the one we were on. I told her maybe she'd better eat another date. She answered in her tone *funeste*, "That was my last one."

I felt a cold sweat spring out under my thermal underwear. The last date! And I no longer had the sugar lump I usually carried in my change purse, because I had unwrapped it two nights before when she was having her *après-ski crise d'insuline*.

(She refused the sugar, of course, electing instead the strange combination of date, peanuts, and crackers, but, anyway, it was unwrapped; so I had left it in our room and had neglected to replace it.) I suggested that maybe we'd better turn around and walk on skis back, especially since we weren't positive the restaurant was open. And, besides, it was still a terribly long up-hill walk.

June demurred, saying we'd walked this far and it would be silly to waste the effort. This didn't comfort me at all. It might just be the manifestation of an oncoming *crise*. When in the early stages of one of these attacks, she gets quite stubborn about what she wants to do. She also likes to observe the *crise* coming on, issuing vague reports about sweating and feeling funny, while stoutly resisting doing anything about it. How did I know but that she was huffing along behind me there, silently observing the symptoms—maybe she didn't recognize the symptoms, especially since one of them is sweating, and who wouldn't be sweating now, even with the gale-force wind blowing?

What would I do if she keeled over? Just leave her there while I skied down for help? How would I describe in French where she was located? And if while I was gone someone found her body, they would naturally assume a ski injury and maybe the phantom (I never had seen one there) ski patrol would take her down the mountain to a receiving hospital and no one would know what was wrong. She didn't have her card or her "I am a diabetic" medal on, and I had neither pencil nor paper with which to leave a note. If she started to go, what could I feed her? Do twigs have carbohydrate? Pine needles?

I couldn't voice any of these fears, because I didn't want her to panic. Panic can bring on all the *crise* symptoms; she would have a false attack. She's had these before when home alone in the bathtub, thinking, "Wouldn't it be terrible if I'm in insulin shock now" and then beginning, at the thought, to feel dizzy, stagger out dripping to the kitchen, wolf something down, and then spill heartily.

I ever so casually suggested that she stay there and watch the skis while I ran up ahead to see how far the restaurant was. She pathetically semi-bleated, "Don't leave me alone here." This really got to me. Obviously, weakness was overtaking her. And I had nothing to offer her to eat. My heart was pounding and I was soaked with sweat. This was my responsibility. She wouldn't even be here if it weren't for me.

I even worried now about skiing back down to the *téléphé-rique* restaurant. We'd gone a good distance and all uphill. If she got on her skis, pointed them down the fall line, and then had an ultimate *crise*, what then?

We rounded a bend in the trail. I could see up above, straight up above, and to the right a lift-keeper's cottage. There was a trail of sunken-in footprints leading up to it. "Look," I said to June, trying not to show my nervous desperation. "I'll just run up the hill to that little place and see how far the restaurant is and try to find out if it's open. I'll be in your sight every minute. You don't have to worry."

And without waiting for an answer I slung down my skis and poles and started running up the hill, trying to match my feet to the footprints, as if I were running a boot-camp obstacle course. I made it to the top, and gasping for breath, staggered over to the shack. I heard a radio playing inside. Encouraged some-what, I rapped on the door. The radio went off. No response. I rapped again. Still nothing. I called out, *"On est ici?"* And since there was still no answer, I pressed the latch, pushed the door open, and looked inside. It resembled the gamekeeper's cottage in a low-budget, realistic, French version of *Lady Chatterley's Lover.*

I called again my *"On est ici?"* Still no answer, so I started looking around for sugar cubes. Apparently this fellow took his coffee straight, for I found none. There was an open cupboard around the corner of the room and to the left. I looked inside and *voilà*, I saw the gentleman's lunch, which included two just about thirds of loaves of French bread, all lovely and oozing carbohydrates. Maybe he'd give me a few scraps of that. I shouted some more and then I went outside and shouted again to no avail.

The platter-pull cogwheel was spinning, and coming up toward me from the vicinity of the restaurant (which looked completely deserted and closed) was a small boy. Even before he was off the platter, I started calling at him in my bad French and asking if the restaurant was open. He didn't understand me and looked a little frightened (I think my desperation had given me a wild Ancient Mariner look).

I was standing in the path of the platter pull when I noticed a woman was coming up. Presumably she was the boy's mother. I started shouting my wild query at her, not noticing in my state that I was right in her path. She was frowning and making negative sounds and gestures at me. I got out of the way just in time, still going over my "Is the restaurant still open?" gambit. "*Je ne sais pas,*" she said curtly as she herded her son away from the mad woman of the mountain.

So there I was without help, without hope, and with a just-about-to-start-fitting diabetic on my hands. I gave a last general shout, waited a second for the non-answer to not come, and then decisively dove into the shed, rounded the corner of the cupboard, grabbed one of the pieces of bread, and ripped out a couple of large chunks. I stuffed these into my parka pocket, tore out the door, and raced down the hill along and over and through and tripping over the footprints in the snow.

I skidded up to June, panting and exhausted, but triumphant. I had by my thievery probably saved her life. I unzipped my pocket and extracted the bread chunks, which I displayed as if they were the crown jewels. June made a face of disgust. "I don't want to eat that junk," she said, "right before lunch."

"*Junk?*" I almost screamed. "What do you mean junk? This is beautiful French bread. It's full of carbohydrates. I stole it for you. Eat it."

She nibbled at a corner, made another face, and put the rest in her pocket. Then she started grousing about why had I been gone so long, did I find out about the restaurant, etc., etc. I explained that no one seemed to know about the restaurant, that it *looked* closed, and it was still a long way, mostly uphill, and if she was going to refuse to eat the lovely bread I had stolen for her, we'd better turn around and go back to the *téléphérique* restaurant. So we strapped on our skis and headed downhill— very slowly, it turned out, because our waxless skis stuck solidly to the wet spring snow every three feet or so.

As we turned a bend in the trail, I looked back over my shoulder and saw a young man in work clothes standing at the top of the hill by the platter pull terminus, hands on hips, gazing steadily down at us. I poled as hard as I could to get out of his sight.

When we reached the restaurant, I confessed to June how terrified I had been that she could have keeled over in the wind and snow and died. She said off-handedly, "Oh, I could always have eaten the candy."

"The candy? What candy?"

"You know, that toffee you gave me that I always carry around in my parka pocket. . . ."

There are, of course, the false attacks that a diabetic sometimes has, but that's not your problem. With a false attack, it's the diabetic who thinks he's going into insulin shock, and he immediately does something about it. Would that June were as conscientious and capable during the real thing as she is during her fits of fancy. She, of course, considers herself eminently sensible and astute about hypoglycemia at all times, pointing out to me haughtily that she has never allowed herself to slip into unconsciousness. My explanation of this is that when she is alone and on her own, she has the intelligence to be much more alert and sensitive to the level of her blood sugar, even doing preventive snacking, than she does in my company, when she can relax and lapse into forgetfulness, knowing I will take over if she starts going goofy.

6. Learn to give the injections.

At this point I can hear the book dropping to the floor from the nerveless fingers of nervous people. Now hear this. There is probably not on the planet a more nervous person than I, especially when it comes to matters physical. I pass out cold and stiff in a doctor's office if he even so much as hints there might be something wrong with me. Yet I managed to overcome and to learn to give June her insulin injection. I guarantee that if I can do it, anyone can, no matter how many white feathers of cowardice he wears in his hat.

It's impossible to believe until you've tried it, I know, but actually it's quite easy, much easier both psychologically and in practice for you than it is for the diabetic himself. And if you have any humanitarian feelings at all, it's a wondrous kind thing to do for a diabetic. It's true that they do start to run out of reachable spots and it's also nice to release them occasionally from the routine. June tells me that when I give her her shot, it goes on behind her back and it's over so quickly that she doesn't even know it's happening. It's almost as if she's not a diabetic for that day. A nondiabetic day is as welcome a present to a diabetic as a handful of emeralds—well, maybe *almost* as welcome.

But like Tom Lehrer's old dope peddler, you can do well by doing good. Cast your insulin into the buttock and it shall come back to you in the form of a resounding injection of self-confidence. The harder it is for you to do the first time, the greater will be your elation when you succeed. That's why I felt so absolutely glorious that first morning at the Ahwahnee when I gave June her fix. I felt my powers were infinite, and as a matter of fact, they rather were. I carried my confidence along with me to the slopes, and I've never skied as well in my life as I did on that day of triumph over chickenosity.

Learning how to give the insulin injection is also important because, when you've mastered that, you've mastered as well the technique of injecting glucagon, the hormone used to revive a diabetic who is unconscious in insulin shock. This could make you a literal lifesaver should you ever encounter a diabetic too far gone to swallow his needed carbohydrates.

But now a warning, Happy though it makes the diabetic to have you give the injection and proud and necessary though it makes you feel, DO NOT DO IT ALL THE TIME. A diabetic has to know how to take care of himself. He can't rely on someone else to always be there. I know a nurse whose husband developed diabetes. She could have given him his shot every day as quickly and easily and painlessly as passing the salt, but despite intense wheedling on his part, she refused with the firmness for which nurses are famous when they're doing something "for your own good."

I also know of an elderly gentleman who has hobbled over to a clinic for his insulin injection every day for the last twenty-five years. I suspect, however, that since he lives alone, the daily insulin trek is as much a way of keeping human contact and combating loneliness as it is of avoiding the personal moment of truth with the needle. But for a normal person with a normal life pattern, it would be a false kindness to make a diabetic as dependent on you as he is on the insulin itself.

7. Don't be too sweet to a diabetic.

I realize that in this book I come off as a devil's advocate, an evil temptress who is forever pushing June toward a glass of schnapps or luring her onto a ski lift or jamming a hunk of carbohydrate down her throat when she least wants it. But that is my duty. Had the diabetic ball bounced in my direction instead of hers, if she is half the friend I think she is, she would be constantly peeling my fingers off the stems of cocktail glasses, snatching Swiss chocolate bars from my lips, and dragging me from the stirrups of a red-eyed, earth-pawing potential skull-cracker of a horse. That would be *her* duty.

For, although Gordon Williams said in *The Man Who Had Power over Women* that it is one of the signs of incipient insanity to divide the world into two categories of people, those who . . . and those who . . . , I do just that. There are those who overdo and those who underdo. I am the former and June the latter. And everyone—man, woman, or child, diabetic or non-diabetic—is either one or the other. Underdoing diabetics have a thinness problem; overdoing diabetics struggle with overweight. Overdoers are the spillers; underdoers are the fitters.

If you have an underdoing diabetic on your hands, you have to keep pushing him lest he make himself into a psychological invalid. If you have an overdoer, you have to continually pull him back before he makes himself into a physical invalid. (Horror note for the overdoers: each year a diabetic is out of control he physically ages five years, and out-of-control diabetes is the leading cause of blindness in women and the second leading cause in men.) About the only thing the overdoers and the underdoers have in common is their lack of gratitude for the pushing or pulling services you perform. More than once June has grown quite churlish at my "bossing her around."

Naturally, if you intend to boss a diabetic around you do have to know what you're talking about. You have to have read and absorbed at least as much on the subject as he, more if possible. You also have to have a doctor to whom you can go for an answer when, as so often happens, the literature lets you down. It's a good idea, if you can, to go to the same doctor as the diabetic. This is because when you have a difference of opinion with the diabetic over what he should be doing, and he asks the doctor to settle the argument and brings the answer back, you may be getting a message as garbled as the ones you get in that whisper-in-the-ear game of telephone.

I recall that when June and I were skiing in Megève, I got very upset with her for refusing to eat a large enough snack in the afternoon. This resulted in a regular five o'clock fit. (Dinner wasn't served in the hotel until 8:00 P.M.) No matter how much I prodded, she wouldn't eat enough to avoid the late afternoon sweats and vagaries. I argued that it was much worse to go into insulin shock daily than it would be to err in the other direction and spill occasionally. (Her idea of being wildly out of control is spilling a more than one-plus every six months.)

When we got back home, I insisted she ask her doctor which was harder on the system, to spill or to shock. She came back with the fuzzy intelligence that "a shock doesn't damage your system." When I went to the same doctor for my physical, I remarked to him that I was suprised that it was no worse for a diabetic to go into insulin shock that it was to spill a little. His jaw dropped stethoscope wards. "Where did you get *that* idea?" I told him it was straight off the June wireless.

"She didn't ask me which is worse," he said. "She just asked if it was very damaging to the system to experience a mild insulin shock occasionally and I said, 'No, not terribly.' But if it's a choice, I'd *much* rather have her spill a little than run the risk of going into a coma."

I can almost hear an overdoer coming home from his doctor and announcing to his family that the doctor said it wouldn't really hurt to have a butterscotch sundae made with chocolate ice cream, neglecting to mention that the end of the sentence was "once every five years."

It's not that diabetics are especially sneaky and deceptive. It's just that they're human. They tend to structure their questions so they get the answers they want. And even when the answer isn't the one they want, they head it that way, anyway.

Another aspect of a diabetic's being human is his tendency to use his diabetes for his own purposes, to get his own way. You can't really blame him. A person is going to fight the life battle with whatever weapons he has available to him, whether they be positive ones like limpid blue eyes or a quick wit or physical grace, or negative ones like being hard of hearing or unnaturally clumsy or, yes, having some malady like diabetes for which he can demand special treatment.

I've seen June use her diabetes to get out of doing what she doesn't want to do, like going to a dull cocktail party. I've seen her avoid foods that aren't to her taste by claiming she can't eat them because of her diabetes. (In this latter case she spreads a lot of misinformation, such as "cucumbers are murder for a diabetic.") She's also apt to claim she has to do something like stay at least two nights in one place on a trip because "changing hotels every day is too upsetting to my diabetes" when it's really just a matter of personal whim. I don't mind her using such ruses with casual acquaintances—we all, diabetic or not, have our own little storehouse of social lies—but I'm determined not to let her get away with such duplicity with me. If you're going to have a healthy give-and-take, day-to-day relationship with a diabetic, you can't treat him as a privileged being who can wave his magic insulin needle in your face and always get his heart's desire.

These problems are all intensified when you have a diabetic child. I've talked to a large number of parents of diabetic children, and from what they say—and even more from what they leave unsaid—I've learned that they suffer from almost universal and massive compulsions to defer to their diabetic tot's every wish and whim. First off, they are consumed by pity. It would break anyone's heart to see a child forever denied the carefree excesses of a normal childhood—the romping to the point of total exhaustion, the gorging on Halloween sweets. It would arouse anyone's compassion to see a child's life depend on being stuck with a needle every day. And when it's your own flesh and blood, it's doubly heartrending and you try to make up his losses with special juicy privileges.

Other parents are gnawed by guilt because they feel they've passed on the genes that make their child diabetic. "I've transmitted this defect to him," they say to themselves accusingly. "It's all my fault." And then they go on to compensate for it to the child in some permissive way or other.

The most tortured parents of all, though, are those who are subconsciously mad at the child for having diabetes. They're upset with themselves for having produced a "defective child," and there he is reminding them of it every day by getting injected with insulin and having to eat a certain diet, a constant living reminder of their biological failure. They're angry and they sublimate their anger by being extra, supercolossally indulgent.

But whatever the motivation, if parents persist in being vassals to their diabetic highchair king, they're bound to turn him into a disaster area of a human being. And if there are other children in the family, their futures are in danger, too. Normal sibling rivalry will blossom into a blooming case of jealousy and hatred, and the nondiabetic children will suffer in their roles of minor planets having to orbit the sun of the diabetic child. A diabetic child is inevitably given more than enough special attention to develop a healthy ego and compensate for what he can't do, which is, incidentally, very little. He shouldn't be given one milligram more attention and consideration than necessary, no matter how good it makes the parent feel at the time.

One legitimate and honest way to make yourself feel better, though, whether you're dealing with a child or adult diabetic, is to allow yourself to get angry with him when he gives you cause. The fact that a person is diabetic doesn't make him immune to doing irritating things, and since you, too, are only human, you should react humanly. For that matter, the diabetic himself should be allowed a natural surge of anger when the occasion calls for it. I know that diabetics are advised to "keep on an even emotional keel," but for whatever my natural-born overdoer's opinion is worth, I believe that emotions are normal and should not be stifled. It's as Huxley said in *Brave New World,* "Men and women must have their adrenals stimulated from time to time. It's one of the conditions of perfect health." Of course, I'm not advocating daily, knock-down, screaming sessions with a diabetic or with anyone else, but neither do I feel it would be a heatlthy emotional climate for a diabetic to dwell in an atmosphere of repressed rage.

And while on the subject of anger, June (and I suppose all the rest of the diabetics who are clever enough to have hit on it) has it set up so she can get angry with impunity. She has a dandy little built-in excuse for any of her acts of distemper. After she has cooled off, she says sweetly and self-justifyingly, "I guess my blood sugar was low."

And here's a final confession for you to match with your own behavior. Sometimes I even get irritated by June's doing something she absolutely has to do as a diabetic. When I'm traveling with her, I don't like not being able to have a brisk, appetite-stimulating walk before meals. When skiing, I resent having to stop in mid-schuss to go find a hunk of carbohydrate. And, worst of all, when we're working on a tight writing deadline and my nerves are like ukulele strings and I'm trying to concentrate and I hear off in the corner the steady chomp-chomp of June consuming one of her relentless snacks, I feel like bellowing, "Cut out that damned chewing or I'll scream."

Of course, I don't do this, or anything else that would bollix up her diabetes, but I *feel* like doing it. And I don't consider myself a heartless monstress for entertaining the thought, and neither should you when your own personal Blue Meanies inevitably rear their ugly heads. After all, diabetics themselves frequently have moments of hating their disease and its restrictions. Many are the times that I've heard June muttering some blasphemy against her body chemistry. Of course, on those occasions when she has had a dramatic drop in her insulin requirements, I've also heard her voicing the quite realistic hope that a period of remission is about to start. Diabetics *do* have remissions, you know. June's insulin dosage has edged down from 20 units to 8, back up again to 14, down again to 10, and so on. We've both become aware that you can never settle back with diabetes and say, "This is the way it is." Tomorrow may be different.

Tomorrow may be better. The research program of the American Diabetes Association is daily getting closer to sniffing out a cure. And to keep their investigative olfactories sharp, it would behoove all of us who are involved with diabetes to put our money where our pancreases are and adopt the ADA, along with our local affiliate, as our favorite charity. Because, although it's certainly true—as I hope June and I have proved in this book—that we can live with diabetes, we can also live without it.

Eighteen years later . . .

Part Two

THE PERIPATETIC
DIABETIC II

Chapter 11

TURNING PRO

A couple of years ago June appeared on the television program "The 700 Club" extolling the merits of self-blood-sugar testing and telling how it had improved her own control. We later heard that a friend who was watching remarked, "It looks as if June's turned into a professional diabetic."

Although this wasn't meant as a compliment, in a sense—a good sense—it's true. During the past eighteen years diabetes has become more and more the center of her life. In the first place she's lived with her own diabetes twenty-four hours a day; in the second, gradually but increasingly we've both started living with other peoples' diabetes. After we wrote the original *Peripatetic Diabetic*, we started receiving letters from diabetics who had questions our book hadn't answered or answers to questions our first book hadn't asked. These formed the core of our second diabetes book, *The Diabetes Question & Answer Book*.

As we came to realize that exercise was the great unsung hero of diabetes control, we researched (both in the library and on location on tennis courts, golf courses, and bike paths) and wrote *The Diabetic's Sports and Exercise Book*. This book put us in contact with hundreds of diabetics of all ages and of all sports enthusiasms who also contributed their experiences.

These books led to invitations to speak to diabetes groups all across the country and to write articles and columns for the various diabetes publications. As a result of the build-up of stresses in our own lives we came to realize the detrimental effects of stress— physical, emotional, and environmental—on diabetes control. Once again we dove into research and personal experimentation until we had the information to write *The Diabetic's Total Health Book*.

About this time we began to receive letters from people who couldn't find our books in their local bookstores and wanted to know where to buy them. The only way we could figure out to solve the problem was to supply the books by mail order. We decided to call ourselves the Sugarfree Center. When people wrote to say they couldn't find diabetes books by other authors, we included some of the best of those in our offerings, too.

The next plea came from people who didn't live near major cities and couldn't find blood-sugar testing strips and blood-letting devices in their local drugstores (some of them didn't even *have* local drugstores). The logical solution was for us to make these supplies available by mail order, keeping the prices as low as possible.

Although our list of products was growing, our staff was just the two of us working off a dining room table. We eventually hired a part-time worker, a young diabetic named Ron Brown, and thus started our reverse discrimination policy of hiring and doing business with diabetics whenever possible. So far, along with our own workers, we've had a diabetic cleaning woman, a diabetic plumber, a diabetic real estate agent, a diabetic insurance broker, and a diabetic who supplies us with carpets and drapes. Around our place Barbara calls herself the "token nondiabetic."

About this time the new blood-sugar testing meters appeared on the market. June managed to get the Ames Glucometer from England before it was available in this country. She was so enthralled with it that we decided to try to supply Glucometers to our local diabetics, and we contacted the Ames Company, which also authorized us to instruct diabetics in meter use.

And now, the Sugarfree Center itself is at last turning pro with a full-time, experienced diabetes teaching nurse and a dietician.

In order to devote our time to writing and working in the Sugarfree Center, we've both taken an early retirement from the library. So you can see how our friend was right with her "professional diabetic" remark.

She was right in another way. June is also a professional diabetic in the sense that after eighteen years she's comfortable with her disease. She feels something the way a professional athlete must. She can play the diabetes game in a relaxed manner because she has the rules down pat. She knows from experience that she can handle the bad breaks and recover from the unexpected. And she strives, like a true pro, to make the difficult appear easy.

What we wish for you is that you, too, become a professional diabetic. We don't necessarily mean that you should make diabetes your life work, although more and more diabetics are. Our first employee, Ron Brown, decided after working with us that he wanted a career in diabetes counseling and has since earned a degree in dietetics at the University of California, Berkeley.

No, what we want you to be is a superstar pro at diabetes, so good at handling yourself that if you were that good in tennis or golf or football or basketball, they'd pay you a million-dollar bonus. As a matter of fact, if you are that good, your bonus will be worth more than a million. It will be the priceless bonus of health.

We hope that the new developments in diabetes therapy and the object lessons we describe in "The Peripatetic Diabetic II" will help you lose your amateur standing once and for all.

Chapter 12

IN SICKNESS
AND IN HEALTH

It was the morning of the eve of June's fifty-ninth birthday—sixteen years A.D. (after diabetes). She was out doing her morning jog. As she rounded the corner and entered the home stretch, she announced triumphantly, "Just imagine. Here I am almost sixty years old, and there is *absolutely nothing wrong with me!*"

Either she had forgotten about diabetes or she didn't consider her chronic disease an impediment to being healthy and in good shape, free from the aches and pains, blubber and decrepitude often associated with age.

Lucky June, right? She's been nothing but the picture of health since her optimistic avowals in *The Peripatetic Diabetic* that the regime imposed on her by diabetes would result in a long and happy life free from major and minor physical complaints. Wrong. In the last eighteen years, the picture of June's health has had a few cracks.

HEADS, YOU LOSE

In 1971, five years after her diabetes was diagnosed, peripatetic as always, we were on a writing-research trip to Cortina, Italy, and Verbier, Switzerland. Flying home, she felt truly miserable: on top of the flu, which she had come down with during the trip, she had also developed a headache—an almost unendurable pain behind the bridge of the nose and the eyeballs that radiated into the forehead.

The flu cleared up, but the headache lingered and lingered. When it finally went away, her relief was short-lived. The head-

130

ache started recurring about 30 percent of her waking hours. Confusing it with a low blood sugar headache, she would try to eat her way out of it, resulting in gigantic spilling of sugar into her urine.

It wasn't surprising that June tried to blame her headaches on diabetes. When you have a chronic disease, you try to lay every physical and emotional complaint you have at its doorstep. But diabetes got a bum rap on that one. The headaches were actually caused by the temporomandibular joint syndrome, a problem with the jaw-hinge joint.

You can read about her experiences in *The Woman's Holistic Headache Relief Book*. But be forewarned—this book isn't the jolly tale that *The Peripatetic Diabetic* is. Although it has a happy ending, it's a chronicle of pain and despair and suicidal feelings that makes dealing with diabetes seem like a romp in the park.

Of course, dealing with diabetes *isn't* a romp in the park, but an experience like June's does provide a little perspective. June always said during her headache days that if someone offered to take away one of her two chronic conditions, she wouldn't hesitate a second. She'd instantly send back the headaches and keep the diabetes. (Apparently somebody was listening.)

So the moral of this tale is that there are worse things than diabetes. But you already knew that. It's just that it's easy to forget. And even when you're philosophical about your diabetes, always nibbling at the back of your mind is the fear of well-known long-range complications of diabetes. That's what June had to deal with next.

A NEUROPATHETIC ADVENTURE

After the headache cure, June regained her former vitality and then some. We took many trips and wrote many books and engaged in many sports activities, and June had many, in fact most, blood sugars in the normal range. She was feeling good, even cocky about her disease and her health. Pride, as always, goeth before a fall.

June was engaged in the extremely nonperipatetic activity of vacuuming. The telephone rang, and, racing to answer it, she managed to trip over the vacuum cord. When she fell, she caught herself with her left hand. The next day her left wrist and thumb joint were painful, but she didn't particularly worry about that until she found the pain was still there the following day and the next.

Barbara, who continues to consider herself one of the great natural uncredentialed physicians, diagnosed the condition as a hairline fracture of the wrist and insisted on whisking the wrist and person attached thereto to the UCLA Medical Center for an X ray. Nothing. Not a crack.

June dismissed the condition from her mind, and the pain subsided. Then one day, when one of our employees didn't show up, she was doing the mail-order packaging in the Sugarfree Center and discovered that when she tried to use any force to close the packages, her left thumb joint became so painful that she couldn't continue the work.

June logically associated the thumb joint pain with the previous injury to the wrist. The thumb pain returned periodically during the next few months, and gradually another problem developed, a numbness in the toes of her left foot. She didn't mention the latter, just noticed it, and, as you can imagine, thought about it a lot. She did, however, continue to complain loud and long about the thumb. It was bad enough that it interfered with work, but it also restricted bike riding—June's all-time favorite sports activity—because the pain in her left thumb joint prevented her from leaning on the handlebars.

Since Barbara couldn't put up with the sound and fury of the complaints, she contacted her own doctor for a referral to an orthopedist. We both thought of the problem as an orthopedic one, induced by the fall, rather than a diabetic one.

When June went to the orthopedist, he had her fill out a long questionnaire. Naturally it came out that she is a diabetic. The doctor commented on the fact as he sent her off to X ray.

When the X-ray photos came back, the doctor inspected them and said, "Just as I suspected. You have diabetic neuropathy."

Diabetic neuropathy?! How could this be? Hadn't June kept her diabetes in meticulous control? Hadn't she exercised? Hadn't she eaten an almost perfect diet? Hadn't she *really tried* to do all the right things? And hadn't we been telling people in our books that if you do all the right things you can avoid complications? But there it was.

The treatment at least didn't involve drugs, which June had come to loathe from her days of taking them to try to zonk her headaches away. She was to put her hands in warm wax twice a day. (She hadn't mentioned the numb toes, or she would have probably been told to put her feet in warm wax as well.) She was also supposed to take massive doses of vitamin B.

From the prescribed treatment, we both got the idea that there isn't really much you can do for neuropathy—except to watch it run its crippling course and try to keep down the pain as much as possible.

We were discouraged, but our discouragement was as nothing compared to that of the two diabetic young women who worked for us. Nanci and Sheila regarded June as a role model. They saw that she took excellent care of herself and as a reward was in great good health. If she could do it, so could they. When they heard that she had diabetic neuropathy it was as if all promises had been broken. If someone like June could develop complications, then why even try?

Gloom reigned in our hearts and minds and filled the Sugarfree Center like a noxious miasma. Was all our work in vain? Was all our writing invalidated?

June began to resign herself to the inevitable. She had a perfectly good Peugeot that had given her reliable service and showed every sign of giving years more of the same. But it was a stick shift. We've both always driven stick shifts because it makes us feel more at one with the car and in better control (in the nondiabetic sense). She went shopping for a car, one with an automatic transmission that she could drive with only one functioning foot and hand if necessary.

Barbara had recently bought a spartan model of the Volvo wagon when her VW flamed out. Since June had driven it a few times and liked it, she turned toward that familiar brand. She was about to get a similar spartan model, except with automatic, when Barbara gently started urging her to get a model with more "conveniences." That is to say, one with such things as windows that you could raise with the press of a button instead of cranking with a (neuropathetic?) hand. June resisted at first, but then, considering her impending decrepitude, she bit the financial bullet and got the luxury model. She liked the car, of course, almost everybody enjoys luxury, but every time she drove it, she was reminded of why she had bought it.

About a month after she bought the car, it was time for her to go to her diabetologist for her regular exam. (She's still with good old Dr. No. 3.) When she saw him, he rhetorically inquired how she'd been getting along, expecting her usual recounting of adventures in good health.

"Not so great," she said, reverting to her tone *funeste*. "You see, I have diabetic neuropathy—here in my thumb and a little in my wrist and I think maybe in my toes, too."

"Let's see," he said, examining her left hand. "There's no reason for you to have neuropathy. You've always been in excellent control."

When he finished his examination he smiled and said, "I don't think you have neuropathy at all. I think you have carpal tunnel syndrome, a wrist problem that causes stiffness and pain. It's true that diabetics are more susceptible to it than nondiabetics, but you definitely do *not* have diabetic neuropathy."

The doctor said that carpal tunnel syndrome can sometimes be corrected with surgery, but he didn't recommend it. He also said that in mild cases, it sometimes just goes away on its own.

Whew! Sighs of echoed relief throughout the San Fernando Valley. June's happiness was only slightly marred by the fact that her thumb still hurt when she tried to package or ride her bike.

Then one day in the letters to the editor section of *Diabetes Care*, she saw a letter, the heading of which caught her eye: "Reversal of the Carpal Tunnel Syndrome After Change of Insulin Injection Sites." The gist was that a twenty-seven-year-old woman with a fourteen-year history of diabetes had stiffness and pain in both hands. She also had lipoatrophy (those indentations you sometimes get from injecting insulin) in her buttocks. Her hand problem was diagnosed as carpal tunnel syndrome, and she was advised to have surgery to correct it. She didn't take the advice.

Later she and her husband were on a trip to California, but neither of them were getting much sleep because of the extreme pain she was suffering in her hands. Probably because he had so many wakeful hours, the husband spent a lot of time thinking. He remembered that the pain in her hands had begun only after the lipoatrophy started developing in her buttocks and that, wishing to avoid this, they had started injecting insulin into her upper arms. They stopped injecting insulin into her upper arms. In ten days the pain and all other carpal tunnel syndrome symptoms went away.

Her doctor, wanting a little more scientific confirmation than this, urged her to start injecting in her arms again to see if the pain would return. She demurred. But finally, four months later, she gave in and started injecting insulin in her arms again. She quit in only two days, however, because the pain returned to her hands. The doctor was never able to persuade her to try again.

We didn't need sleepless nights to get the idea and make the connection with June's problem. Whenever we went out to dinner together, something we increasingly did because neither of us had time to cook, Barbara usually drove, in case June's blood sugar might do a preprandial plummet. When we got to the restaurant and parked, June would bare her left arm and ask Nurse Jane Fuzzy-Wuzzy to give her an injection there. Always it was the *left* arm because Barbara was always sitting in the driver's seat and that was the one she could reach.

We stopped doing this, and, sure enough, the carpal tunnel syndrome cleared up completely. June keeps saying that in the interest of science she's going to inject in her arm again to see if the pain comes back, but it's been more than a year now, and somehow she hasn't managed to get around to it.

And what of the toes? Nothing of the toes. The numbness is gone, and no pain has come in to take its place. The toes are just toes again.

This tale has a couple of morals. First, be suspicious if a doctor who is not your regular physician tells you a condition is caused by your diabetes when he or she hasn't even ascertained what kind of control you're in, and for something as significant as diabetic neuropathy always get a second opinion and always get it right away so you don't have to writhe around building up tension and stress over what could be nothing.

Second, before you go out and spend a bunch of money on

something to make life easier for you in your physical deterioration, be sure you really are deteriorating—unless, of course, you need an excuse to spend a bunch of money on something you want anyway.

THE EYES HAVE IT

Now that it no longer reminded her of her "diabetic neuropathy," June grew wildly fond of her new Volvo. It nearly broke her heart when, even before the new car smell had dispersed, she backed into a post in an underground parking structure and bashed in the right rear fender—a $480 dent.

The accident forced her to acknowledge something she had been pushing to the back of her mind. She just wasn't seeing very well out of her right eye. It was cloudy going on murky. She was fairly certain it wasn't retinopathy, since she'd been given such a clean bill of microvascular health from her diabetologist only a few months before. She suspected a cataract. She was right.

The ophthalmologist told her it was a very fast-growing variety. That's why her problems with the eye, including the post bashing, had come on so suddenly. He said he'd operate just as soon as there was an opening in his schedule. (Three months later!)

June had read that diabetics are particularly susceptible to cataracts, so she asked if her diabetes had brought this on. "Oh, no," the doctor said with warm reassurance. "This isn't a *diabetic* cataract. This is a *senile* cataract."

So for the next three months every time June told anyone about her impending operation for her cataract, she'd announce with pride, "It has nothing to do with diabetes. It's a *senile* cataract."

Because of June's diabetes ("You never know what might happen with a diabetic"), she couldn't have the surgery in the doctor's office the way many of his other patients did. She had to check in at the hospital the night before and have the surgery the next morning.

Despite all the horror stories we'd heard of diabetes not being handled correctly in hospitals, we were sanguine about the event. After all, this was one of the best hospitals in the Los Angeles area.

They'd know how to take care of things. No problem. We decided to relax and make something of a party of it.

Barbara delivered June to the hospital and then went out for an order of sushi to munch on (and fill the room with the vapors of). When she returned to the room, June was already in high huff. "They wouldn't let me take my insulin!"

"You mean they're going to make you eat dinner without insulin?"

"No, I mean they wouldn't let me take *my* insulin. They said it's against the hospital rules for patients to administer their own medication. I have to send my insulin home with you, and they gave me *this*." June's insulin was purified pork. *This* was not. *This* was also ice-cold and foamy. *This* had been taken straight from the pharmacy refrigerator and sent up via the pneumatic tube.

At least they let her take her own blood sugar since that's not considered a medication. And a good thing, too. The hospital had no diabetes care nurse, and no one seemed at all familiar with self-blood-sugar testing meters. When June asked what they do when they have newly diagnosed diabetics in the hospital, one nurse told her, "They show them a film."

The worst was yet to come. June could have no breakfast before surgery. (Remember what happened to the patient in *The Verdict*.) Therefore, she drew back in horror when the nurse approached her at 6:30 A.M. with a syringe and the rechilled insulin. "Oh, no! You're not going to give me that!"

"Oh, yes," she replied, drawing the insulin into the syringe. "Doctor's orders."

"What doctor?"

"Your surgeon. Your dose of insulin is four units of Regular and four of Ultralente." (This is what June had written down as her usual morning insulin schedule on her preoperation questionnaire.)

"But not when I'm going without eating. If you give me that, I'll go into insulin shock and die on the operating table." June isn't above using slight hyperbole when right is on her side. But then something decidedly unpleasant *could* have happened if she hadn't fiercely stood her ground.

The nurse finally gave in to the irascible recalcitrant and went off to try to call the doctor for permission to omit the injection. Apparently she got it because she never returned.

The surgery was routine, so routine that June, who had a local anesthetic, recalls that the group huddled around the operating table were discussing the merits of a condominium purchase.

Meanwhile, back in June's room, Barbara was pacing around wondering what had become of her. The surgery had been scheduled for nine o'clock, and time passed and passed and passed until it was after one. Where was she? Had there been complications? Was she up there connected to some kind of life support system while surgeons pounded on her chest trying to get her heart started again?

No, not exactly. She was in the recovery room, recovered to the extent that she was bright and alert and furious and ranting. "When is somebody taking me back to my room? I haven't had any insulin for eighteen hours. My blood sugar must be soaring. Why can't I go back to my room and take my insulin?"

They tried to placate her and explain that they were shorthanded and most of the orderlies were still at lunch and just as soon as another one came on duty, etc., etc.

The fuming June arrived in her room about a quarter to two, loudly demanding her insulin. A nurse came in and reported that they couldn't find her insulin and so had to send down for another cold and foamy one. June had taken her blood sugar and realized that she needed more than her normal dose of regular to get back to normal so she requested several additional units. No. She was to get her usual noon dose and that was that. June started to rant again until Barbara gave her a "cool it" look as the nurse went off to see if the insulin had arrived yet.

"Just let her give you what she wants. I still have your insulin in my purse. You can take whatever you want after she leaves."

The nurse was amazed at June's sudden docility.

June loaded up on insulin and waited for her lunch, which the nurse said would be forthcoming. It did not forthcome. Barbara kept padding down the hall, nagging and whining about where was the lunch and it's almost three and she hasn't eaten since dinner last night and she's starving and she's full of insulin. Time passed. June was reaching for the glucose tablets, and Barbara was preparing to run down to the cafeteria personally to get June lunch, when the door crashed open and a nurse June had become acquainted with the day before came skidding in with a big glass of orange juice. She had just come on duty, and after looking at June's records realized she'd had her insulin (little did she know how much) but nothing to eat. June had drunk most of the orange juice when the lunch finally arrived. Since she was starving she ate most of the lunch and a combination of the juice and the food and the stress sent her blood sugar soaring.

June demanded to go home.

"But you're scheduled to stay another night."

"I'm going home."

"But since you stayed past one o'clock, you'll have to pay for tonight anyway."

"I don't care. I'm going home. I'll pay anything to get out of here." (Spoken like a true person with good insurance coverage.)

"But I'll have to get permission from the doctor to release you."

"Do it."

She did it and June escaped, leaving behind the reputation of being the scourge of the fifth floor—make that the scourge of the west wing or maybe even the whole hospital.

The moral of this is obvious, but just to hammer it home here's an excerpt from the excellent book *Diabetes: A New Guide to Healthier Living for Parents, Children and Young Adults Who Have Insulin-Dependent Diabetes,* by Lee Ducat and Sherry Cohen:

CAN YOU TRUST THEM AT THE HOSPITAL?
No!

Once again, it's a question of being your own best advocate. When you have a chronic disease that's so misunderstood and so replete with myths, *you probably know more than almost anyone else about your day-to-day care*. And you have to insist upon your right to exercise that care as you've learned is best for you.

So plan ahead—as June didn't. If you understand your diabetes and keep yourself in good control and if you'll be in condition to take care of yourself, ask your diabetologist to make arrangements for you to handle your own diabetes while you're in the hospital.

And if they're doing something to you that you know is wrong, become the scourge of the floor or the wing or even the whole hospital—as June did.

THE SUMMING UP: TOTAL HEALTH

At least June's hospital experience ended well. The cataract is gone, the lens implant works perfectly, and she's never crumpled another fender.

Back before Richard K. Bernstein had written his *Diabetes: The GlucograF Method of Normalizing Blood Sugar*, and before he added M.D. to his name, he used to write us to announce his increasingly ideal blood-chemistry figures, among other health statistics, resulting from his program of self-therapy. He said we were probably the only people he knew who were interested. Maybe nobody's interested in June's figures (except maybe Dr. Bernstein), but we feel they are significant if you want to see how her health fares after eighteen years of diabetes.

Height: 5'5"
Weight: 110
Resting pulse: 68
Blood pressure: 127/70
Cholesterol: 182
Triglycerides: 79
Hemoglobin alc: 8.2

In fact, here she is sixty-one years old, and there's *absolutely nothing wrong with her*.

(Barbara's numbers are just as good. In fact, in her last physical her doctor told her she had the blood chemistry of a twenty year old. She attributes this to eating and exercising as if she were a diabetic. Tell that to your nondiabetic family members and friends!)

June is the first one to admit that a lot of her success is due to good luck. She's lucky her genes didn't program her for any disease on top of diabetes. She's lucky that all the new therapies and tools for staying in control came along during her diabetes lifetime so she could take advantage of them. She's lucky that she loves exercise and always has, so following a regular sports and exercise program is not a chore for her but a joy. She's lucky that she's never been hung up on food—especially desserts and sweets—so the dietary restrictions have never been a hardship. (Barbara says that since June's not all that interested in food, she doesn't deserve a lot of credit for her abstemious eating habits—any more than a person with a low sex drive deserves a lot of credit for moral behavior.)

But she's worked at it, too, and we're convinced that almost every diabetic with a little bit of luck plus work and perseverance can say, "Here I am _____ years old, and there's *absolutely nothing wrong with me.*" We've been criticized a couple of times for dispensing all this encouraging word. One person said we tend to make people who have complications feel guilty, feel that they didn't do enough to prevent them. That was never our intention. We know that some people had diabetes before the current therapies were available and that they didn't have the tools for good control. They couldn't help it. We also know that some people try as hard as they can, yet still have problems with their diabetes. It's not their fault. But for most diabetics today we feel, along with Dr. Bernstein, that "diabetes doesn't cause complications. Poor therapy causes complications." And we want to do everything in our power to help you do everything in your power to have good therapy and prevent complications.

What do you need for this good therapy? First off you need a good Dr. No. 3–like physician, then you need a lot of learning (a lot of learning is a safe thing), and, finally, you need a certain amount of sweat, a few occasional tears, and you need blood—yes, as you'll read in the next chapter, you definitely need blood.

Chapter 13

BLOOD SISTERS

If we ever do a roots search, we both suspect that we'll find we have Transylvanian antecedents going all the way back to Count Dracula, so passionately enthusiastic are we about self-blood-sugar testing.

We first discovered this key to good control back in the summer of 1975, when we were writing *The Diabetic's Sports and Exercise Book*. Among the 158 diabetic sportspeople who corresponded with us, sharing their ideas and experiences, was a young man who said he checked his blood sugar with Dextrostix before heavy sports activity. Dextrostix?! What are *they*?

Not long after that we saw a reference to them in an article on travel for diabetics by Dr. Stanley Mirsky in *Diabetes Forecast*. Dr. Mirsky advised that the diabetic's travel companions carry the "stix" so that in case the diabetic was found unconscious they would be prepared to determine quickly whether the cause was hypoglycemia or hyperglycemia. The way it worked was that you put a drop of blood from your fingertip or ear lobe on the chemical reagent pad on the end of the Dextrostix. After a minute you washed off the blood and compared the color of the reagent pad to a chart on the side of the strip container. The paler the color, the lower your blood sugar; the darker the color, the higher your blood sugar.

Since this kind of test seemed perfect for diabetic sportspeople —in fact, for diabetic all-kinds-of-people—we set out to find some Dextrostix to experiment with. After checking with several pharmacies, we finally had to special order them. Pharmacists, at least in our area, didn't regularly stock Dextrostix, and many seemed quite vague as to what they were.

When we got the strips, June jabbed her finger with an old

insulin needle (ouch!), got the drop of blood, put it on the pad, washed it off, and read it. Correction, *tried* to read it. It was very difficult to determine (guess) the blood sugar by comparing the murky purple of the pad on the strip to the murky purple of the color chart on the vial of strips. Therefore, we were delighted to learn that there was a meter, called an Eyetone Reflectance meter, that could read the strips for you. When you inserted the strip into the meter, a needle on a dial would point to the number (in milligrams) of your blood sugar.

We called up the local Ames Company representative to see if we could borrow one of these meters to carry out our experiments for the book. Since the meters cost around $600 in those days, June didn't feel like taking the financial plunge for one without knowing how—or even if—it worked. We did manage to borrow one, and June started taking her blood sugars with it.

June had always thought that she was in good control because her semiannual blood sugars at the doctor's office were invariably normal. (Of course, she was always extra careful with her eating on the days of the tests. That's only the human thing to do.) But besides that, the urine tests that she did several times every day hardly ever showed sugar.

When June read her blood sugars on the meter, though, she was surprised, even shocked, to find that they were frequently over 200 and sometimes even hit the 300 range. Although she didn't know what to call it at the time, what she had was a high renal threshold. She didn't spill sugar in her urine until she was over 200. This frequently is the case with diabetics over the age of forty, and it's a good reason why diabetics in that age group should test their blood sugar rather than their urine even if they don't take insulin.

One thing June did know, and know right away, was that her old urine tests weren't telling her what was going on. Along with not telling her when she was high, they also couldn't tell her when she was low. (She found occasional 30s and 40s registering on the meter when she'd been exercising and hadn't eaten enough.)

June decided she had to have a meter. Luckily, she was able to get a used one for $350. We never could figure out why someone was willing to give up such a delectable instrument. Another thing we couldn't figure out was why these strips and this meter weren't loudly and widely advertised as the diabetic salvation that they were. One regional manager, who is no longer with the company, told us in confidence (never tell us anything in confidence!) that most physicians were violently opposed to having their diabetic patients test their own blood sugar and the company didn't want to alienate the doctors—who used a number of other products it made—by promoting their self-blood-sugar-testing line.

We immediately took it upon ourselves to promote the strips and meter whenever possible in books, in articles, in lectures, and even in casual conversations. Other diabetics, notably Richard K. Bernstein, were out there assiduously doing the same. A grass roots self-blood-sugar-testing movement started sprouting all over the country. As diabetics became aware of the possibilities of testing their own blood sugar, they "jumped on it like a duck on a june bug," as John A. Owen, Jr., M.D., graphically put it in his outspoken article, "Ars Longa, Ars Nova (Or, Can We Monitor Self-Monitoring Patients?)," which appeared in the May 1981 issue of *Modern Medicine*. This article was aimed at his fellow physicians and urged them to face several facts about self-blood-sugar testing:

1. Patients, not physicians, have found a new approach to diabetes.
2. Patients, not physicians, can now control diabetes superbly.
3. The technique is easily mastered by anyone (regardless of education), the end results look promising, and patients are overwhelmingly delighted.

He then invited physicians to face some difficult to answer questions: "Would we be so cautious and skeptical [about self-blood-sugar testing] if this innovation had been introduced by a physician, and concerned a new technique for physicians to use? Can we tolerate a doctor-patient relationship in which the patient learns more about his disease than we do? And if we are willing to give it a try, what will be the nature of the new relationship, the new state of the art of medicine?"

Times they gradually did begin a-changing. The drug companies realized that there were a lot of diabetic ducks there hungry for self-blood-sugar-testing june bugs, and they finally decided to supply—and advertise—them.

One of the most welcome developments was the introduction of the Autolet, a little device to get the blood out of the finger easily and almost painlessly. June's blood-sugar-testing frequency almost doubled when she could use that instead of used insulin needles or hand-held lancets. In pre-Autolet days, she would usually kind of peck at her finger with the needle or the lancet, not breaking the skin, and then finally in disgust plunge in, releasing a Texas gusher. After the pioneering work by the company that makes the Autolet, other companies came out with the Autoclix, the Hemalet, the Penlet, the Monojector, and Auto-Lancet. A bloodletter for every taste (as we latter-day Draculas would put it) and every pocketbook.

Bio-Dynamics had introduced its easier-to-read, tough and stable Chemstrip for visual reading in 1979, and the diabetic grassrooters were cheering for it. Ames developed two new meters: first the Dextrometer and then the Glucometer, and it also got on the visual-strip bandwagon with the Visidex and, a couple of years later, the improved (no wash!) Visidex II.

Bio-Dynamics came up with the Stat-Tek meter and later the Accu-Chek. The Glucoscan meter arrived from England, and then its American importer, Lifescan, created its own all-new Glucoscan II. Orange Medical Instruments brought over another British meter, the BetaScan. Still another meter from England, the Glucochek II, was distributed and later bought out by Larken Industries in Kansas. Ulster Scientific, the company that first introduced the Autolet to America, released its new meter, the Glucokey.

Wouldn't it be nice if some company named its meter Arthur or Edna? Trying to keep all this "chek" and "gluco" stuff straight is enough to drive you crazy and raise your blood sugar. To help alleviate some of the confusion about which meter does what and how it does it, we've prepared "The Sugarfree Center Unscientific and Opinionated Report on Meters" (see Appendix C).

In the fall of 1983 a wonderful thing happened for diabetics. Increased competition brought on the Great Meter War. Some meter prices dropped to as low as $150, bringing meters into almost every diabetic's realm of possibility, especially since most insurance companies and even Medicare were at last willing to pay a percentage of the cost. They finally realized that meters bring good control and good control keeps diabetics out of the hospital and thereby saves the companies and/or the government piles of money.

And, speaking of saving money, Larken Industries developed a strip cutter and a narrower track to put in their Glucochek II meter, making it possible to read a half-strip in a meter. (Clever diabetics had for years been cutting their Chemstrips in half or even in thirds for visual reading.)

You can see from all this that there are now enough self-blood-sugar-testing june bugs available to fill an entomological museum as well as the craw of every diabetic duck. And what is more important, most physicians have become true believers in self-blood-sugar testing. The diabetologists led the way, and almost all the others have followed their lead. We say *almost* all the others because an incident that happened only a few months ago made us realize that there's still a lot of missionary work to do out there in Doctorland.

Barbara was standing in line at the bank behind a uniformed nurse. Never wanting to miss an opportunity for a little medical talk with a fellow Nurse Jane Fuzzy-Wuzzy, she inquired whether the nurse worked in a hospital or a doctor's office.

"A doctor's office."

"Oh, is your doctor some kind of specialist?"

"No, he's a general practitioner."

"Do you have many diabetic patients?"

"Lots of them!"

"I guess you have all of them doing self-blood-sugar testing."

"Oh, no, we don't do *that!*" she said, making a face as if Barbara had asked whether they taste their patients' urine for sugar.

This is the sort of thing that inspires us to keep banging the drum loudly in favor of blood-sugar testing and dinging the gong loudly against urine testing, except for ketones when blood sugars are running high or when the diabetic is ill or has an infection.

We may have been banging and dinging a little too loudly. We even went so far as to announce in the *Health-O-Gram*, the Sugar-free Center's newsletter, that we didn't even stock urine-testing supplies except for ketone testing.

An irate reader immediately fired back an anonymous postcard bearing the following message: "Apparently you're not interested in diabetic children. *You've* decided, quite arbitrarily, not to stock urine-testing equipment, but you've never tried testing the blood of a small child on a three or four time a day basis."

Not surprisingly this communiqué disturbed us and set us thinking. We consulted our medical advisers for the *Health-O-Gram*, the Guthries (Richard Guthrie, M.D., and Diana Guthrie, R.N., Ed.S., F.A.A.N., C., of the Kansas Regional Diabetes Center in Wichita). They said that in their studies with young children, the Clinitest two-drop method correlates quite well with hemoglobin A_1C tests.(The test shows overall control for a three-month period.) They also pointed out that children's fingers *are* smaller, and there's less space for repeated punctures.

In the next issue we reported this and also that we were now stocking Clinitest in the Sugarfree Center.

Almost by return mail we received this impassioned plea from a mother and fellow Dracula descendent:

Please continue to urge blood testing! I'm the parent of a three-and-a-half-year-old diabetic who was diagnosed at twelve months of age. We've done home blood testing for the last year. It was like coming out of the dark ages. No more watching for dilated pupils and beads of sweat, no more guessing whether or not it is a temper tantrum or hypoglycemia.

More important, we used to experience middle of the night "howling" and seizuring episodes. It is a horrifying experience that requires fifteen to twenty minutes to subside. . . . Now I can put my son to bed with a 120 or higher blood sugar and be confident that he and I will be able to sleep through the night without a hypoglycemia episode.

When I talk to other parents I make it clear that the younger the child is, the *more important* it is to do home blood-glucose testing. Children cannot tell you how they feel. Just last week my son's urine test before bedtime was 2 percent plus, yet his blood sugar was 54!

I do at least four blood tests daily on little fingers. I know parents of tiny infants who invert the platform on the Autolet to get as little penetration as possible.

Back we went to the Guthries, who, in great part, agree with this mother, but since this blood-sugar testing versus urine testing is such a complex issue, they were kind enough to write a complete report on their recommendations (see Appendix H).

For the majority of diabetics, self-blood-sugar testing is inevitable and will eventually do wonders for all diabetics' control as it's done for June's. Her records aren't perfect, but they are a far, far better thing than they were back when she had her first experiences with the old Eyetone Reflectance meter. She does sneak over 200 occasionally and once in a very great while scratches at the door of 300. When she is high, she doesn't stay that way very long because with her insulin schedule, she can bring her blood sugar down again right away.

This brings us to an important point that we haven't emphasized enough. (You *can't* emphasize it enough.) Self-blood-sugar testing is not an end in itself. You don't test your blood sugar and then say, "Nice blood sugar there" or "That's a pretty bad blood sugar" and then go your way. Self-blood-sugar testing is a tool to get good control. It tells you when you've done something right, and it tells you when you have to make changes. You take your records to your doctor, and he or she then works out a program (diet, exercise, insulin, medication, etc.) with you that keeps your blood sugar in the normal range as often as possible.

Using her meter as a guide, instead of the old insulin schedule she used in *The Peripatetic Diabetic* (a single shot of 10 units of NPH before breakfast), June now usually takes 4 units of Regular and 4 units of Ultralente before breakfast, 2 or 3 units of Regular before lunch, and 3 units of Regular and 4 units of Ultralente before dinner. This plan is a modification of the one Dr. Bernstein uses in his GlucograF method. It is sometimes called "the poor man's pump" since the Ultralente is a long-range (thirty-six-hour), almost nonpeaking insulin that provides a basal rate the way the insulin infusion pumps do and the Regular insulin is used to cover meals—like "bolusing" with a pump.

June has not yet tried a pump. She feels she is doing as well with her conventional method of three shots and four or five blood sugars a day as she would with a pump. In fact, some studies have shown that you can do as well. However, if you're interested in improving your control with a pump, we suggest you write for a free subscription to *Pumpers*, 2 Woods Chapel, Rolling Meadows, IL 60008, a magazine for information-sharing among pump users.

The meter also makes it possible for June to know whether she should increase or decrease her Regular insulin before meals or take insulin supplements when she's sick or has an infection and her blood sugar gets out of control.

Incidentally, June's insulin is Nordisk purified pork and Lilly Iletin I beef/pork Ultralente. No manufacturer is yet making Ultralente purified pork, which is now recommended over the beef/pork mixture as it builds fewer antibodies. She is holding off on trying the new human insulin, made from recombinant DNA technology or made from the conversion of pork insulin, until more diabetics have reported their results and until it is available in Ultralente. Human insulin peaks faster, has a shorter duration of action, and causes fewer antibodies than even purified pork. Meanwhile, we can all rejoice that synthetic insulins mean that no matter how many diabetics there are there will always be enough insulin for all.

Another important use of the meter is to tell you when your blood sugar is low and you need to take something to bring it up again. This takes us to a question June is frequently asked: Has she ever passed out with hypoglycemia? No, she hasn't, but she's had such low blood sugar that it brought on such obnoxious behavior that those around her—especially Barbara—almost wished she *would* pass out.

One time June was starting to act a little peculiarly. She seemed vague and disoriented. Barbara suggested that she take something since she appeared to have low blood sugar.

June bared her fangs and snarled, "I do *not* have low blood sugar, and I'm sick of having you always say that I do."

Barbara cleverly realized that she was, indeed, low and dropping fast, so she quickly got the package of Destrosols (glucose tablets), took out three, held them out to June, and said, "Here, eat these."

June recoiled in horror. "I won't take those from your filthy, stinking hands. Your hands stink. Do you know that? They *stink*. In fact, *you* stink. Get away from me. I can't stand the smell."

Although she knew June was in the throes of low blood sugar, Barbara was baffled. "Do my hands really smell bad? Have I been cutting garlic or working in the garden and forgotten to wash my hands?" She sniffed her fingertips while June cowered in the corner trying to get away. No, there was no garlic or any other smell that she could ascertain. She cautiously approached June and said in a placating way, "Now, you really *have* to eat these," and put the tablets in her hand. June hurled them across the room. "I won't eat those stinking things out of your stinking hands!"

Barbara tried to stick a Dextrosol into her mouth. June clenched her teeth against it.

"Either you eat this, or I'm going to inject you with glucagon."

"I won't let you. I won't let you touch me with your stinking hands."

"Okay, then I'm calling the paramedics. *They'll* inject you with glucagon."

Somehow that threat got through the hypoglycemia barrier, and June, making a face, took a Dextrosol and slowly, reluctantly started chewing it. After two more Dextrosols and a half glass of orange juice, she became herself again—a self that never uses words such as *stink*.

The other memorable hypoglycemia event took place in our publisher's office. Although it is memorable, neither of us remembers it—probably we've repressed it as one tends to do with embarrassing moments. Our editor, Janice Gallagher, however, loves to remind us of the occasion.

We were having an editorial conference on *The Woman's Holistic Headache Relief Book* with Janice and the publisher. There were a lot of problems to work out—problems that would involve our doing a great deal more work. Time passed as we tossed the problems back and forth. Janice remembers that June gradually grew silent and just sat there staring at the floor and glowering. Although Janice knew that June was a diabetic, she didn't really know anything about diabetes and how it can sometimes affect a person's behavior.

Barbara was so absorbed in the "exchange of ideas" (argument?) that she didn't notice that it was well past June's lunchtime, nor did she notice June's silence.

When it appeared that the discussion was over and the course of action agreed upon, Barbara turned to June and said, "Well, I think we can make those changes and get the manuscript back in about two weeks. Don't you think that's okay, June?"

June looked up at Barbara and barked out a two-word obscenity. Janice's jaw dropped.

Although Barbara had never before (or since!) heard June utter this phrase, especially not directed at her, Barbara didn't miss a beat. She looked around the room at the amazed faces and asked matter-of-factly, "Does anyone have any raisins or something we can give June?"

Janice recalls that this amazed her even more. "If someone said something like that to *me*," she thought, "I certainly wouldn't be offering them raisins."

Despite these near misses, June has never passed out. But Barbara has. Isn't this carrying being a *diabétique imaginaire* a little too far? Yes, definitely.

Barbara has this little problem with hyperventilating. Whenever something threatens her well-being, even if she just thinks she's going to be sick to her stomach, the anxiety causes her to breathe rapidly, too much carbon dioxide leaves her system, and she passes out. While she's unconscious her breathing returns to normal, and after a few minutes she regains consciousness. It's not what you'd call a serious condition, but it can be inconvenient, not to mention that it scares the wits out of those about her.

One Saturday we were scheduled to speak at a large diabetes conference at California State University, Northridge. Barbara felt she was coming down with the flu, but that didn't stop her from doing her morning jog, which, as any sensible person could have told her, made her feel a hundred times worse.

The eminent Los Angeles diabetologist Leona Miller was giving the keynote address before we were to break up into smaller conference groups. Barbara was guarding Dr. Miller's purse and taking notes when she began to feel really bad and as if she might soon be really sick. She didn't want to create a scene in the lecture hall, so she tottered past June and out the back door.

The next thing June remembers was someone bursting through the back door, shouting, "Is there a doctor in the house? [Actually

there were about twenty of them.] A diabetic has passed out."
June, realizing what had happened, ran out the door to find the
unconscious Barbara flat out on the floor. People were running
around hysterically shouting for orange juice. June, who by now
takes Barbara's hyperventilation events calmly, figured she was being taken care of, and since Dr. Miller was making some important
points she didn't want to miss she returned to the lecture. (Always
the pragmatist.)

The next thing Barbara remembers was swimming into consciousness and finding a doctor cradling her head holding a glass of
orange juice to her lips.

"I don't need that. I'm not a diabetic," she said as stubbornly as
any diabetic in the throes of hypoglycemia would. The doctor per-
sisted, and, when Barbara realized that the only way she could get
up and go about the business of the day was to capitulate, she
drank down the whole glass. Thus fortified, she managed to get
through the two lectures. Between lectures the major topic of conversation was "A diabetic woman passed out" and "I wonder if she's
all right" and "Did they send her to the hospital?"

A few more events like that and we'll be able to write *The
Peripatetic Hyperventilator* and Barbara will at long last get to have
top billing on the book jacket.

Chapter 14

PORTRAIT OF THE DIABETIC
AS JACK SPRATT

Have you ever looked back on an old boyfriend (or girlfriend) with whom you were desperately enamored and wondered, "Whatever could I have seen in him/her?" That's the way we now feel about fat. How could we have carried on the way we did about such a miserable substance—and its first cousin, grease, is even worse. And carbohydrate, about which we wrote so disparagingly and condemned as the enemy of diabetic control, how could we have been so unfair, and wrong? Ah, well, we were younger then, but it wasn't totally our youth and inexperience that led us astray.

Phyllis Crapo, R.D., an expert in nutritional research, recently wrote in *Science* that we're just beginning "to pull nutrition out of the dark ages." So we were in the dark ages then and just as unenlightened as everybody else. We thought of fat almost as "free" for June. Since she was the opposite of overweight, fat could do her no harm. She could use fat to fill out her plate that had to be so restricted by the dread carbohydrate.

Our enlightenment began when we were trying to cure June's headaches. Since diet is sometimes implicated in chronic headaches, we started reading in the area of nutrition and paying more attention to what we were eating. The more we read and researched, the more reasons we found for cutting back on fats—they cause a rise in cholesterol and triglycerides, which contribute to the cardiovascular problems diabetics are particularly susceptible to, animal fat is frequently a storehouse of chemicals from pesticides and pollution, fat is increasingly being implicated in cancer of the breast and colon, and, of course, for those who do have to worry about excess pounds, fat puts on weight since it has more than twice the calories per gram as protein and carbohydrate.

153

This turned us in a new dietary direction, and Dr. James Anderson, of the University of Kentucky and author of *Diabetes: A Practical Guide to Healthy Living*, started us down the path of nutritional righteousness. He found that his HCF (high carbohydrate and fiber, low fat) diet often reduced insulin dose or eliminated the need for oral hypoglycemic pills. This is because, as he said, "for many diabetics the fat in their diet is their worst enemy. Eating fat blocks the action of insulin—the body cannot burn sugar very well after a meal containing a lot of fat."

Dr. Anderson also found that complex carbohydrates such as those in beans and whole grains and vegetables were good for diabetics, actually serving to level out their blood sugar. His book thoroughly explains this diet and gives the special exchange lists for following it. We reprinted Dr. Anderson's exchanges in our *Diabetic's Total Health Book*.

So June changed her alliances. She now recoiled from fat, her former friend, and cozied up to carbohydrates. While she didn't completely embrace the HCF diet—mainly because she didn't have the time to cook up the piles of grains and pots of beans that being a total HCF follower would require—this diet made a profound change in her dietary habits.

The American Diabetes Association made some changes in its exchange lists, too. In 1976 it issued a new, lower fat version. The meat exchanges are divided into "Lean Meat," "Medium-Fat Meat," and "High-Fat Meat." (A copy of the A.D.A. exchange list is available from the American Diabetes Association, 2 Park Avenue, New York, NY 10016 [write for current price]. It is also reprinted in the appendix of our *Diabetic's Total Health Book*.)

Gradually the whole dietary world started turning around. In 1977, the United States Senate Committee on Nutrition recommended that in order to reduce the death toll from heart attacks, strokes, and diabetes, all Americans should make the following diet changes:

Increase consumption of vegetables and whole grains.
Decrease the use of sugar and foods high in sugar.
Decrease fat and cholesterol by cutting back on meat, eggs, and high-fat dairy products.

Eat more poultry and fish, and drink nonfat milk.
Cut down on salt and salty foods.

So, it turned out that what's good for diabetics is good for the
nation. And, strangely enough, not just our nation but even
France. France, the home of everything swimming in a sauce
awash with cream. France, where there are as many cheeses as
there are days in the year and where most of these cheeses actually
boast on their labels of how *high* the fat content is. France, where
the rillettes, pâtés, and terrines are literally packed in pork fat or
goose grease. France, where they even put butter on radishes.

Led by famous French chefs such as Paul Bocuse and Michel
Guérard, the *nouvelle cuisine* and *cuisine minceur* started empha-
sizing fresh vegetables and eliminating heavy sauces. The plates
also were garnished in an artistic way so that the eye appeal was as
great as the gastronomic appeal.

This movement quickly spread to the increasingly health-con-
scious United States. Restaurants featuring young, creative new
chefs—and creative new higher prices—sprung up right in our own
backyard. (The less expensive, family-style French restaurants
didn't pick up on this movement, continuing to serve their sauces
and butters and cream as in days of yore.) So you see, it turns out
that after all these years, we continue to relish those times when
we can afford to eat in Very Expensive French Restaurants at home
and abroad, and June continues to do very well with her diabetes
in them. That is, *most* of the time. . . .

We always go out to dinner to "celebrate" June's diabetes anni-
versary, March 17. It's kind of a way to beat the devil. At any rate,
since it's such a special occasion, we always try to go to a really nice
place—usually a Very Expensive French Restaurant.

Several people had recommended to us that we try a new
French restaurant in Los Angeles. We had also read that one of
the best features of this restaurant was that it always
served three fresh vegetables with the entree. That's our kind
of place.

It was a small restaurant on Sunset Boulevard, decorated with
what you'd call tasteful restraint, unless you call it stark. The menu
featured a lot of imaginative-sounding fish dishes and a number of

veal (a notoriously lean meat) dishes. Right on the diet! Everything, incidentally, was à la carte.

We started with a Very Expensive Green Salad. It arrived. It
had about seven leaves of lettuce (but who's counting?) and a couple of leaves of radicchio (the new, chic green, which is actually
red, popular in southern California restaurants these days). It was
lightly coated with a delicate, nonoily dressing. Nice, but at that
price we felt maybe we could have had, say, fourteen leaves of
lettuce, four leaves of radicchio, and perhaps even a bit of endive.
Ah, well, no one wants to fill up on salad when there's a wonderful
entree coming garnished with three (three!) fresh vegetables.

Our entrees arrived. June's veal medallion was about the size
(and thickness) of a piece of Monopoly money. Barbara's fillet of
fish was so small it would probably have been rejected as bait by a
fisherman. But what of the vegetables? We did get three fresh
vegetables, didn't we? Right. We each got three vegetables: one
green bean, one cauliflower floweret, and one miniature carrot,
very artistically arranged on the plate. During the meal we kept
stuffing down bread, the only edible in adequate supply, but we
were still starved when we finished. There was no choice but for
each of us to have a dessert, something neither of us generally
does. Barbara had a strawberry tarte, June an apple one. The desserts were the only courses that were served in generous measure,
and we were both so hungry that we almost licked the platter
clean.

We won't tell you what the bill was because we try not to put
depressing information in our books, but it was enough to buy the
new Prince tennis racket that Barbara had been longing for but that
she felt was too expensive.

But the *colmo*, as they say in Spanish, was that if June were still
using Tes-Tape, it would have been as green as ever it was on her
day of diagnosis. As it was, her meter gave her a thumping 300.

We must admit that the Los Angeles Very Expensive French
Restaurant scene has improved in that no longer is the fare quite as
minceur as it was, possibly in response to the furious letters people
wrote to Los Angeles restaurant critics about having to stop off for
a Big Mac on the way home from such restaurants.

Another wonderful development in major American cities is the rise of the Very Expensive Italian Restaurant. These usually feature the lighter northern Italian cuisine, which seems to have a French chef's touch.

There's one major reason we've been more and more often leaning across the Italian gastronomic border: pasta. June can eat twice as much pasta without raising her blood sugar as she can bread (even whole wheat bread) or rice or potatoes. We were very puzzled as to why this should be until, in the spring of 1983, we heard about a new breakthrough in carbohydrate research for diabetics.

As it usually happens in diabetes reporting, the newspapers got hold of the breakthrough and blew it all out of proportion, spreading a lot of misinformation in the process.

You may remember such headlines as "Diabetics Can Eat Sugar." From what they went on to say in the articles, a casual reader might infer that it's now okay for diabetics to eat piles of sugar and mounds of ice cream. That, of course, is a lot of baloney (to name another nonrecommended dietary commodity).

In the first place, *nobody*, diabetic or not, should eat piles of sugar and mounds of ice cream. In the second place, the research was done on such small numbers of people—thirty-five or so—that it would be premature, even foolhardy to make drastic changes in your diet based on what are only preliminary findings.

What basically happened—and is happening—is that scientists are now testing to see how individual foods affect blood sugar. One of the leading researchers in the area, Dr. David Jenkins of the University of Toronto, has created a new classification of carbohydrate foods. It's called the Glycemic Index. What it is is a gauge of how fast and high certain foods raise blood sugar.

Generally speaking, for diabetics a low (slow-releasing) Glycemic Index food is preferred to a high (fast-releasing) Glycemic Index food. The following chart shows the Glycemic Index of some of the few foods that have been tested.

CARBOHYDRATE GLYCEMIC INDEX

Simple Sugars

Fructose—20

Sucrose—59

Honey—87

Glucose—100

Fruits

Apples—39
Oranges—40
Orange juice—46

Bananas—62
Raisins—64

Starchy Vegetables

Sweet potatoes—48
Yams—51
Beets—64
White potatoes—70

Instant potatoes—80
Carrots—92
Parsnips—97

Dairy Products

Skim milk—32
Whole milk—34

Ice cream—36
Yogurt—35

Legumes

Soybeans—15
Lentils—29
Kidney beans—29
Black-eyed peas—33

Garbanzos—36
Lima beans—36
Baked beans—40
Frozen peas—51

Pasta, Corn, Rice, Bread

Whole wheat pasta—42
White pasta—50
Sweet corn—59
Brown rice—66

White bread—69
Whole wheat
  bread—72
White rice—72

Breakfast Cereals

Oatmeal—49
All-Bran—51
Swiss Muesli—66

Shredded wheat—67
Cornflakes—80

Miscellaneous

Peanuts—13
Sausages—28
Fish sticks—38
Tomato soup—38

Sponge cake—46
Potato chips—51
Mars bars—68

As you can see from glancing over this chart, the new findings are often surprising:

> Some foods previously thought to cause a fast rise in blood sugar cause only a gradual rise (apples, ice cream).
> Some foods thought to cause a gradual rise are really fast releasing (shredded wheat, carrots, potatoes: "Potatoes are like candy to a diabetic.")
> Fructose (in controlled diabetics) causes less blood sugar increase than other simple sugars (only 20 percent as much as glucose).
> Legumes (beans, peas, etc.) cause slow rises in blood sugar.

Dr. Jenkins warns, however, that blood sugar is only one factor to consider in diet. You have to figure calories and nutritional values as well. As things now stand a diabetic cannot and should not eat by the Glycemic Index alone—especially since so far there are only sixty-two foods listed on it and, as June says, "Some of them— like Mars bars and potato chips—I wouldn't touch with a ten-foot tongue."

But June welcomes the arrival of the Glycemic Index because, at least for her, it seems to work. And anything that gives you a built-in excuse to refuse parsnips has to have something going for it. (Please don't write to us, Amalgamated League of Parsnip Farmers. We were only kidding.)

The index also explains a few things that used to confuse us. We never could understand why the carrot puree favored by a number of our Los Angeles restaurants *always* caused June's blood sugar to shoot up. We suspected that they must be putting sugar in it, although they swore they weren't, but when June stuck Tes-Tape in the puree, it invariably turned green. (See, there's still some use for that former mainstay of June's life.) The Glycemic Index would also seem to partially explain the success of Dr. Anderson's HCF diet, since so many of his recommended foods have low index numbers.

While we wait eagerly for more research to be carried out and for more additions to the index, we personally intend to:

1. Eat more pasta and legumes.
2. Remember that although ice cream may be low on the index, it is high in fat and calories and must be measured and counted in the diet.
3. When dining out and there's a choice on the menu, go for the lower index food. For example, choose sweet potatoes or yams over white potatoes.
4. Use fructose for cooking and some sweetening, but do not use it wantonly. It has as many calories as sugar.

While we're on the subject of sweeteners, we've had a lot of questions lately about aspartame (trade name NutraSweet). Aspartame is a combination of two amino acids, aspartic acid and phenylalanine. (Yum!) When you put them together they make a clean sweet flavor without an unpleasant aftertaste. So far it appears to be safe for most people, although it must be avoided by anyone with the genetic disease phenylketonuria (PKU). That eminent medical organ, *The Wall Street Journal,* also warns that "one researcher has said a combination of aspartame and carbohydrate— a diet drink eaten with a sandwich, for instance—could affect brain chemistry and behavior." NutraSweet is 200 times sweeter than sugar and has only 2 calories per teaspoon in its table form (Equal).

Beatrice Trum Hunter devotes several pages to aspartame in her book, *The Sugar Trap,* and voices a number of objections to its use, including the PKU warning. Mainly, however, she feels that not enough tests were done before it was allowed on the market. Of course, Beatrice Trum Hunter basically objects to all sweeteners, both artificial and natural. And, to tell the truth, so do we. We feel it's better to get rid of your taste for sweets totally.

We're also realists, though, and know that most people do enjoy a sweet taste and will get it one way or another. (We read in one anthropological study that the craving for sweets was programmed into us back in our monkey days to encourage us to swing over and grab a piece of fruit off a tree so we'd get the necessary vitamin C in the diet.) We'll also confess that, sugar-free saints though we are, we have to put some sweetening into the Always on Friday Muffins (see Appendix A), and we sprinkle a little Equal into our espresso.

If you want to use artificial sweeteners of any kind and drink soft drinks sweetened with artificial sweeteners, we recommend using the "Rule of Two" suggested by our Sugarfree Learning Center dietician, Barbara Recio. Limit yourself to two packets of artificial sweetener per day, or you could make that one pack of sweetener and one artificially sweetened soft drink. The Rule of Two definitely doesn't mean you can have two packs of sweetener, two soft drinks, two artificially sweetened puddings, etc., a day until you've built yourself up to the point of one gentleman whose wife stopped by the Sugarfree Center and asked if we thought he might be overdoing the NutraSweet a bit since he was using fifty packs a day.

Although we know we'd all be better off using no artificial sweeteners at all, we think the Rule of Two is a good way to establish the outer limits.

You can use the Rule of Two in other areas in which you're seeking moderation for health or even financial reasons. For example, since, as we mentioned in the introduction, truffles have now gone up to $38.00 an ounce, you might also want to limit yourself to two of those a day—or maybe a lifetime!

Chapter 15

PEREGRINE
AND BEAR IT

In a certain limited circle, Barbara's mother has garnered herself quite a reputation as an etiologist—one who studies the origins of diseases. Her particular area of discovery and expertise is the "travel disease." She first isolated and nomenclated it once when we were telling her that a mutual friend was going on her second trip to China. Barbara's mother shook her head and with a look of sorrow said, "It looks as if she has the travel disease."

On another occasion when we mentioned that another friend was going to Paris for a couple of weeks, she looked amazed and disgusted, making, as the French would say, a *moue*. "Why would he want to go *there*?" After a musing pause, she answered her own question. "I guess he just has the travel disease."

It's not surprising that she should specialize in the recognition and study of this condition, since her own bewildering offspring has been a victim of it since the age of twenty-two. June, too, has had this chronic condition for a long time—many years longer than she's had her other chronic condition.

Look at the number of flare-ups of the travel disease we've had in the last eighteen years. There were trips to Guadalajara and Budapest and Saint John's and Quebec and Hong Kong and Cleveland. There were trips to Singapore and Bora Bora and Prague and Vancouver and Stockholm and Wichita. There were trips to Aspen and East and West Berlin and Bruges and Sri Lanka and Leningrad and Omaha. There were trips to St. Paul de Vence and Arnhem and Oslo and Rome and Papeete and Missoula. And, as the travel brochures are wont to say, much, much more. In all of these travels June never got sick. Never? Well, hardly ever. She did get ill

162

for about three days from eating fish in Cleveland. And then there was Sri Lanka. . . .

Sri Lanka, which means "resplendent isle," used to be called Ceylon. It's the small island nation off the tip of India. For this reason it's sometimes called the "tear drop of India." Actually this is a strange anomaly since Sri Lanka is in a sense India *without* tears. While it's far from a wealthy nation, you don't see the soul-grinding poverty that you do in its larger northern neighbor.

Sri Lanka is famous for tea, gemstones, spices, teak, exotic birds, elephants, monkeys, and beaches with sand like soft brown (you should excuse the expression) sugar. It's also renowned for its Buddhist shrines such as the Temple of the Tooth, which contains a tooth of the Buddha, and the 2,200-year-old Sacred Bo Tree, which is a sapling from the Bodhi tree under which the Buddha received Enlightenment.

And thereby hangs the tale of why we hied ourselves off to spend two weeks on this small morsel of real estate literally on the other side of the world. June, as we mentioned before, has been studying Buddhism. In Sri Lanka, Buddhism has been preserved in its purest form for almost twenty-five centuries. She therefore decided that she would make a pilgrimage there to celebrate and commemorate her early retirement from the Valley College Library and her new total focus on diabetes education.

So she planned and we read. Barbara, who is usually quite sanguine and never worries about travel mishaps, began to grow uneasy as she read about cobras and cholera, malaria and typhoid. She'd heard of people who went to India—just a few miles across the water—and developed terrible kinds of dysentery. They almost died. What would a disease like that do to a diabetic? Possibly remove the word *almost* from the sentence? She began to say things to June like, "Are you sure you *really* want to go to Sri Lanka? Wouldn't you rather go to Spain or Greece or Norway or . . . ?"

No. June was insistent. Sri Lanka it had to be.

So Sri Lanka it was. And it was, indeed, a rougher kind of travel than we'd ever experienced. The food was usually a curry of unrecognizable ingredients, except for the chili pepper that was all too easy to recognize, and some of the accommodations weren't exactly AAA approved, and the heat and humidity were often oppressive and enervating. Still June had no problems at all. She glowed with good health and good spirits.

We planned to spend the last few days in Sri Lanka at the Mount Lavinia Hotel, a semi-luxury establishment on the Indian Ocean. We wanted to relax and swim and get ready for the long flight home.

On the last night the hotel had a giant outdoor fish barbecue. You were to walk along a large buffet table, select your fish (raw!), and take it to one of the charcoal broilers where it would be grilled for you. That was the theory. In practice the logistics didn't work out. There were too many people to handle in this way, and, as the crowds milled around, the unscrupulous among us, not wanting to· wait, cut in and made off with fish being grilled for others. This happened to us a couple of times, and June, already beginning to feel her preprandial insulin, began to get restive. In desperation we grabbed our third try for fish off the grill before it was done, and since that was the only protein available, we ate it.

In the early dawn of the next morning, Barbara began to feel the unmistakable stomach cramps of the classic malady of tourism. She headed toward the bathroom, turned on the light, and looked toward the object of her trek. She didn't have her contact lenses in, so what she *thought* she saw was a kind of furry Roto-Rooter coming up out of the toilet, kind of thrashing around as if someone in the next room had been cleaning out the drain and the cleansing device had taken a wrong turn into this plumbing.

She looked closer. Even without her lenses she could perceive that the thing was alive, but she couldn't figure out exactly what the thing was. It appeared to be long and skinny. Thinking fast, Barbara remembered that the two creatures you're most likely to see in Sri Lanka are cobras and mongeese (mongooses?).

"June," she shouted. "Quick! Call the front desk and tell them that we've either got a cobra or a mongoose in the toilet."

Although June is not famous for doing what she's told without question, this time she groggily complied.

The person on duty seemed baffled by June's report but assured her someone would be there right away to see what was wrong.

Back in the bedroom we both cowered as far from the bathroom as possible, listening to the water splashing, and expecting the creature from the porcelain lagoon to come slithering out the door at any minute.

After forever there was a knock at the door. We admitted two uniformed men—they looked like security guards. One was carrying a broom. They entered the bathroom as we resumed the cowering position.

We heard shouts, bashing and crashing, and then something fast and low and hairy streaked out the door and down the hall with the broom-wielding attendant in fresh hot pursuit and the other right behind him.

In only a couple of minutes they were back laughing heartily. (Sri Lankans have a great sense of humor!) The creature was a rat, one of the men reported and, still laughing, measured from his elbow to the tip of his middle finger to indicate its size. They went about their business, leaving us to our packing and our musing on the morning's event.

The first musing was the interesting fact that Barbara's incipient disease had been instantly cleared up by the creature encounter. The second musing was why the attendants had just chased the rat down the hall and had apparently done nothing to exterminate it permanently. June's theory was that since Sri Lanka is primarily a Buddhist nation and Buddhists don't believe in killing anything, they just let the rat run free. Barbara's theory was that they were just trying to be helpful. There were no doubt other tourists staying in the hotel who might have developed an inconvenient malady from the fish barbecue, and they were shooing this living, nondrug combination of Lomotil and Kaopectate into one of their rooms to effect another miracle cure.

On the flight out of Sri Lanka, alas, the malady hit June, and, since there was no rat in the plane's lavatory, nor in our Hong Kong hotel room, she was forced to suffer with it for several days. We don't know if she was spilling ketones or not because we had forgotten to pack the Ketostix. (Always carry all diabetes and medical supplies you might need on a trip. Don't do as we do, do as we say.)

But she survived it all, and now, just as with birth pains, the problems fade from memory while still vivid are the thoughts of the smiling—sometimes laughing—friendly Buddhist people of Sri

Lanka; the blood warm waters of the Indian Ocean; the Hindu and Buddhist *poojas* (religious ceremonies) complete with banging drums, wailing horns, and swirling incense; the elephants giving themselves trunk-squirt showers in the rivers or being gently prodded into work by their *mahouts;* the monkeys jungle-gyming through the trees; the parakeet fly-by we observed while floating on our backs in a pool in Anuradhapura; the giant statues of the Buddha in the medieval capital of Polonnaruwa; and June's most cherished memory, the saffron-robbed diabetic monk at Mount Lavinia who insisted on running back to his room to get his Orinase tablets to show her. (Ah, the family of diabetics!)

Despite all of its wonders, we're not necessarily urging you to go to Sri Lanka. We're urging you to go to the place you want most to experience for your own special reasons and to not let your diabetes—or fearful friends and family members—stop you.

AIR FARE

When you do travel by air, we're displeased to report, the food situation is the same as it was eighteen years ago. We agree totally with Ted Willke, editor of *Pumpers*, who recently reported in that magazine, "The only thing worse than airline food is the special diabetic meal. Twice . . . I ordered special meals ahead of time. Instead of being served first, I had to wait for the other 283 passengers to be served. I sweated and waited, all the time being assured that my food would arrive. By the time it arrived, it was cold and tasteless especially after three candies. The only thing dietetic was the extra portion of fruit and the noticeable lack of salt so generously used on the regular meals. I now take my chances with the other passengers."

In a valiant attempt to update our old list of what airlines serve diabetics (an appendix in the original *Peripatetic Diabetic*), we wrote to every airline that has offices in the United States. The only answers we received were from Frontier, Lufthansa, and American Airlines. (If they have to cut back on personnel in the financial crunch, it's better that they cut back on P.R. people who might answer our letters than on mechanics who maintain the planes!) At any rate, our best advice is always brown bag it on airlines. As usual, we don't always follow our own best advice. June usually just takes the regular meal. Barbara usually tries for something different: vegetarian, kosher, children's (hamburger or hot dog and hold the junior stewardess wings), and sometimes even diabetic.

ARRHYTHMIA AND BLUES

After all our years of time-zone-crossing travel we're still plagued with jet lag or its more technical term, arrhythmia. It's unlike any other body sensation. Your whole biological time clock is out of sync, you're disoriented, exhausted, and dopey during the day, and as alert as a rabbit in the middle of the night, when you're trying to go to sleep. You don't feel at all like yourself, and it takes almost a day for every hour of time zone change you've been through for you to feel normal again.

Since jet lag, just like any other strain on the body, can affect diabetes adversely, and since the strange body signals can sometimes mask—or masquerade as—low blood-sugar episodes, we've continued to be particularly alert for new ways to counteract this problem.

Dr. Karl Neumann, a Forest Hills, New York, pediatrician and travel writer, came up with a dandy one: when you fly to and from Europe, always fly on the Concorde. He says that flying at supersonic speeds (1,400 mph) both gets you there faster and allows "your mind and body to resume normal efficiency sooner than after flights on conventional jets."

One of the reasons for jet lag symptoms is that the air conditioning on a plane gradually removes all the moisture from the air. This lack of humidity fatigues you and makes an uncomfortable dry feeling in the mouth, eyes, and skin and may even be a factor in causing feet to swell. The body can endure about four hours of this treatment (the length of time the SST flight takes) without too much ill effect, but over that the trouble begins.

The cabin pressure of the SST is better too—the equivalent to being on a mountain at around 4,000 feet—while a conventional jet is more like 6,000 feet. "That difference of about 2,000 feet," Dr. Neumann explains, "means that aboard the SST you have fewer problems with your ears and less intestinal discomfort from expanding gas."

The better pressure also means you'll have more oxygen to breathe and, again, have less fatigue and be less affected by the carbon monoxide from cigarette smoke that by the end of a flight fills the whole plane including the no-smoking section.

And then there's the ozone that in a conventional plane, Dr. Neumann points out, can cause "a burning sensation in the eyes, a dry feeling in the mouth and throat, and sometimes a hacking cough. . . . The presence of ozone reduces oxygen in the blood. This puts a slightly greater burden on the heart and lungs." In the SST, the air intake valves are located next to the engine where the heat destroys the ozone before it can get into the plane.

Coming back from Europe, the SST is even better for avoiding fatigue and jet lag. Conventional jets take almost two hours longer returning than they did going because they're bucking west-to-east jet-stream winds, whereas on the SST the flight time is the same both directions because it's above the jet stream.

It's above something else, too. The price of an SST flight from New York to London is $2,094, and from London to New York it's $2,258.

Thanks a lot, doctor. Great idea you have there.

Moving right along, we come to a new theory espoused by Dr. Charles Ehret, a chronobiologist with the Argonne National Laboratory, who believes that what you eat is the most important factor in offsetting the effects of jet lag. Based on this theory he's developed the Argonne Anti-Jet-Lag Diet. This diet calls for a four-day, preflight regimen of alternate days of feasting and fasting. On the feast days, you eat a high-protein breakfast and lunch and a high-carbohydrate dinner (including a dessert). On fast days you eat as little as possible, and what you eat should be low in carbohydrates and calories (for example, light soups and salads, fruit, and unbuttered half pieces of bread).

Since the whole idea of the diabetic diet is to eat approximately the same amount every day and not to fast if you're insulin dependent, just what this doctor orders is not right for diabetics. But if you have intellectual curiosity about what the diet entails or if you have family members who want to try it, it's written up in the book *Overcoming Jet Lag,* by Dr. Charles Ehret and Lynne Waller Scanlon (Berkley Books, 200 Madison Avenue, New York, NY 10016, $4.95). You can also get instructions on the diet by writing the Argonne National Laboratory, 9700 South Cass Avenue, Argonne, IL 60439.

So it pretty much looks as if we're still stuck with our own, old, familiar, moderately successful jet lag avoidance routines: try to start adjusting to the new time zone a few days before you leave by getting up an hour earlier each day (if you're flying east to west) or an hour later (if you're flying west to east). Don't get into a frenzy of activity before you leave and take off in a state of exhaustion. Sit on the aisle if you can so you can get up and walk around the plane every hour if you're not sleeping. Each time you take your walk, also drink a large glass (or several small paper cups) of water to counteract dehydration. Drink no alcohol of any kind. (One experienced traveler believes that jet lag is one-half hangover because the altitude increases the effect of the alcohol; alcohol is also dehydrating.) Eat lightly, preferably from a bag of food you've brought along yourself that contains things that are just right for you. This way you can eat it when you need it and not when it occurs to the cabin staff to serve it.

If you're flying to Europe from the West Coast of the United States or to Asia from the East Coast, try to break your trip and stay a night or two in an American city on the opposite coast from yours. If possible, schedule your flight so you arrive at your ultimate destination in the evening and can go to bed within a few hours. Take it easy the first few days so as not to further stress an already stressed body. Change your watch immediately to the new time zone so you aren't always checking to see what time it "really is." This is psychologically bad because, for example, you'll immediately feel sleepy if you know it's 2 A.M. back home.

Stay relaxed, knowing that, while jet lag may be bothersome, it isn't critical or chronic, unlike the travel disease, which is both. Incidentally, just in case you really get sick or have an accident while you're traveling in this country or abroad, it's a good idea to sign up with one of the emergency services listed in Appendix D.

You might want to write to all of them for information and select the one that suits your needs best. It usually turns out that if you're prepared for everything, nothing happens, so be prepared.

THIS SPORTING LIFE

Actually we prefer to think of travel not as a disease but as more of a positive addiction. It's not the only positive we're addicted to. Sports comes in a close second—or maybe even it's a tie. Of course the best of all possible worlds is a sports vacation, and since last we've met in Peripatetic Land, we've picked up a few new sports to vacation with.

For us one of the best ways to get out from under stress is to get next to a natural body of water. For that reason we took up surf fishing and found there's nothing like standing there on the beach with the water foaming over your bare feet, casting out to where the waves break, feeling the tug of the receding tide—and the occasional jerk of a fish on the line or, more often, stealing the bait. You don't stand there pondering your problems or monitoring your blood sugar. You stand there with a gloriously blank mind. It's probably a similar feeling to transcendental meditation.

An even deeper meditation state comes from actually getting into the water floating face down wearing a mask, hypnotized by the slow rhythm of your breath in the snorkeling tube and the sight of the coral formations and the tropical fish so vivid and varied that you feel you've invaded a Beverly Hills psychiatrist's office aquarium. When you really need to relax, this is it. Whether you do it in the Pacific area (Hawaii, or French Polynesia), where you fall into a state they call "Polynesian paralysis," or in the West Indies, where it might be named "Caribbean catatonia," you feel something shut down inside you. It's the great adrenaline machine that back in so-called civilization keeps pumping out the blood-sugar-raising stress juice day after day after day until it seems a normal way of life. If you're an insulin taker, be prepared for your requirements to drop along with the tensions. That, after all, is what a vacation's for.

Vacations are also for vigorous activities, and we do still try to do our share of those. In the last few we've mostly given up downhill skiing in favor of cross-country. Cross-country is more aerobic, and we're always looking for ways to tone up the old cardiovascular system. If you don't wander off and get lost in the wilderness, it's also a lot safer. In downhill we didn't ever worry much about hurting ourselves, but over the years the out-of-control skiers on the slopes seem to increase geometrically. After you've heard a few screechings in your ear, "Get outta my way! I can't turn these things," or, June's favorite, "Look out, lady, I'm gonna get you!" you begin to seek less hazardous experiences on the X-C trail.

But our true favorite sports vacation activity is biking. June, even back in her prediabetes days, always had a dream. She wanted to take a bicycle tour of Europe. She talked about it for years. For one reason or another—time, money, responsibilities, commitments—she kept not doing it. Time passed. She became, as the French delicately put it, of *un certain age*. (Indelicately put, fifty-seven.)

Then one day we saw in the paper that the Netherlands National Tourist Office was offering a Holiday on Two Wheels, a group of "All-in (!) cycle package tours for small groups and individuals."

We investigated and found that there were more than a dozen tours to choose from and they were indeed "all-in," including breakfast, dinner, lodging, and the use of a bicycle. They also provided extremely detailed directions on how to get from here to there the most scenic way possible.

It seemed that this was the ideal opportunity and the ideal time —now or never—for June to finally realize her postponed dream. We selected two tours. The first was an Arnhem Boomerang Tour. This meant you stayed in one hotel for three nights and biked around the woodsy Arnhem area each day. We thought this would be a good way to get our bike legs in shape. It was. It was also a way to get used to our bicycles, which, though they were shiny and new, were not lightweight ten-speeds, but rather forty-pound one-speeders. Luckily, Holland is as flat as the proverbial pancake, which must have been invented there since you find so many places serving up *pannekoeken*.

After that warm-up, we came face to face with the reality of June's dream in the form of a seven-day Two Provinces Tour. We stuffed all our belongings for a week into the two saddlebags that hung across the back of the bikes and pedaled off.

Each day we had to cover a certain number of miles, sometimes as many as fifty, to get to the next hotel in time for dinner. After fifty miles on the bike, June ate as if diabetes had never entered her body or mind. And though the dinners were set menus, she never worried about straying from her diabetic diet since the meals provided were always wholesome and balanced, and included lots of vegetables. Best of all—even after nightly plate cleaning—June always stayed in control. In fact, her daily insulin needs dropped from 18 units to 10.

The diabetic body, we found, thrives on this kind of daily regime. But it is as nothing compared to what happens to the diabetic spirit. It soars. It sings. Hey, you're really doing it! And it's better than the dreams ever were or could be. You're skimming along special bike paths through the woods ("Did you see that little red fox? That deer? Those baby wild boars?"), along the tops of dikes, past slowly turning windmills and farmhouses set back from the road and surrounded with flowers.

And the silence. You can actually hear a cow tearing off a mouthful of grass as you ride by. Your city-congested sinuses open up. An elderly Dutch couple cycle past. You can smell the pipe tobacco smoke that clings to his tweed coat and the scent of her cologne. You sleep as if zonked by the most powerful of narcotics. You awake restored and eager to ride out your dream on your natural high for another thirty to fifty miles.

How about *your* prize dream? Now's the time to wake up and start realizing it with no diabetic excuses.

What do you do after your dream comes true? Why you quickly get yourself another. June's new dream was to celebrate her sixtieth birthday by riding the number of miles of her age and, three years later, bike it she did in a coastal area north of Los Angeles. Nothing to it.

Next new dream: to golf her age. From the way her golf game's going, in order to do that she'll have to live to be the oldest woman on the face of the earth. We'll let you know how her dream's working out eighteen years from now.

Part Three

THE DIABETIC REFERENCE BOOK: APPENDIXES

A CHEW OF OUR
FAVORITE THINGS:
COOKING AND DINING

When we first published *The Peripatetic Diabetic* the idea of *haute cuisine* for diabetics was totally bizarre. The diabetic diet was a prosaic and boring *basse cuisine*—which could also be spelled *bah! cuisine*. Because we couldn't stand the thought, to say nothing of the food, we took all the culinary tricks and treats that we'd picked up in cooking classes at the University of California Extension and the Cordon Bleu in Paris, in our travels, and in experiments in our own kitchens and created our own diabetes recipes. These we put into a minicookbook in part two of the book.

Happily, in the intervening years the entire world of diabetes cooking has made a turn for the better. The difference in the diet then and now is like the difference between food in a high school cafeteria and at Faugeron, our favorite Parisian V.E.F.R. (Very Expensive French Restaurant).

This wonderful change was brought about by imaginative dieticians who showed patients how to break out of the old dining patterns and indulge in food that not only is exciting but also suits perfectly their lifestyles and ethnic preferences.

And with the new cookbooks in hand, every diabetic and his or her family can create and enjoy dishes that are as delicious as they are healthy for everyone. Here are a few of our favorites:

The Art of Cooking for the Diabetic, by Katherine Middleton and Mary Abbot Hess (Contemporary Books, $8.95). This most complete, creative, and informative diabetic food and recipe guide is the perfect launching pad into new culinary orbits. Good, sound tips on everything from nondairy creamers to wines in cooking. There are 300 fully calculated recipes personally perfected by a diabetic counselor and a nutrition educator with diabetic family members. Emphasizes low saturated fat and low sodium.

The Calculating Cook, More Calculated Cooking, Diet for a Happy Heart, Fabulous Fiber Cookbook, Secrets of Salt-Free Cooking, by Jeanne Jones (101 Productions, $6.95 each). The author, herself a diabetic and a gourmet cook, has combined her experience and talents to produce five excellent cookbooks that help you stay on your diet and make dining a joy. The first two are specifically for diabetics, but since Jones has such a feeling for the needs of diabetics, all the recipes in every book have the exchanges figured.

Sugarfree Microwavery Calculated Cookbook, Sugarfree Kid's Cookery, Sugarfree Sweets and Treats, by Judith Majors (Apple Press; *Microwavery* $6.95, others $4.95 each). This author is also a diabetic and one who confesses that she "lives to eat." These three books happily help diabetics do both. *Microwavery* has 140 of her favorite recipes that you can cook quickly and easily and fat-freeily in your microwave. *Kid's Cookery* is a collection of calculated recipes that have child appeal and that are simple enough for a young diabetic to prepare. As you know, we're pretty hard-nosed about sweets and encourage you to try to lose your taste for them entirely. However, we realize that while you're coming down off sugar, you may need some sweets to taper off with and on special occasions you may want to give yourself a treat. *Sugarfree Sweets and Treats* can help you meet these needs and wants. All of Major's recipes here are sweetened with fruit and fruit juices—no sugar or artificial sweeteners. All three of these books are A.D.A. Oregon Affiliate approved.

Francine Prince's Gourmet Recipes for Diabetics, by (you guessed it!) Francine Prince (Simon and Schuster, $9.95). We've tried a lot of diabetic cookbooks that purport to be that overused word *gourmet*. At last we've found one that lives up to the title. Here are 175 original recipes that are exciting, imaginative, quick, and easy. Another plus is that they're minus sugar and salt and high in fiber. (We particularly relish her gumbo.) Prince is our kind of cook, and since she invites readers to write and ask questions she's our kind of person as well.

Oriental Cooking for the Diabetic, by Dorothy Revell, R.D. (Japan Publications, distributed by Harper and Row, $9.95). Dr.

Ee-Chuan Khoo, who wrote the foreword to this book, put it well: "Mrs. Revell has served up a delicious collection of recipes, tempting to the Oriental as well as to the sophisticated Occidental palate. She has managed to combine the scientific principles of Western diabetic diets with the exotic ingredients of Eastern cooking. She has made life more interesting for the diabetics of both hemispheres." This includes both Chinese and Japanese recipes along with a smattering from other Oriental countries. A welcome breakthrough in exotic dining for the diabetic!

Light Style: The New American Cuisine, by Rose Dosti, Deborah Kidushim, and Mark Wolke (Harper and Row, $8.95). More than 250 delicious low-calorie, low-cholesterol, low-fat, and low-salt recipes, each followed by a dietary analysis and diabetic exchanges. The sweeteners used are mainly fructose or fruit. We so loved these recipes that we included the one for lasagne in our *Diabetic's Book: All Your Questions Answered* to prove that food can be low in fat and calories and perfect for the diabetic diet, yet can still be a wonderfully complex and savory concoction worthy of the table at a V.E.I.R. (Very Expensive Italian Restaurant). These same authors have also published *Light Style Desserts,* so if you haven't quite pulled out the old sweet tooth with Judy Major's help, you might want to check that out as well.

Laurel's Kitchen, by Laurel Robertson, Carol Flinders, and Bronwen Godfrey (Nilgiri Press, $18.00; Bantam, $4.95). This isn't strictly a diabetic cookbook in that it doesn't have the exchanges listed for each dish, but for the diabetic who wants to be a vegetarian or who simply wants to eat a more healthful diet, it's a vital guide. If we had to choose and say one cookbook is our favorite, this would have to be it. The philosophy is beautiful, the recipes are delicious and wholesome (in the best sense of the word), and the scientific information is totally accurate and totally understandable. Whenever we feel low physically or emotionally, we turn to *Laurel's Kitchen*—and we have the feeling that if we followed its edicts all the time, we'd feel low less often. Get the paperback, and then when you fall in love with it, get the hardcover to live with forever.

Exchanges for All Occasions, by Marion Franz, R.D., M.S. (International Diabetes Center, $7.95). In the original *Peripatetic*

Diabetic, along with our recipes, we also included an expanded exchange list to show that diabetics can eat on the exchange system yet not be stuck with the paltry few items listed on the sheet given to you along with your diagnosis. We moved the exchanges forward an inch; Marion Franz has advanced them a mile. There are more than 450 foods listed according to exchanges. All the popular mystery foods are here: fortune cookies (3 equals 1 bread), kiwis (2 equals 1 fruit), granola bars (1 bread and 1 fat). The only staple of our diet that we found missing was French crescents (*croissants*). We called Ms. Franz, and she instantly supplied it: 1 crescent equals 2 breads and 2 fats. There are special lists for high fiber, vegetarian, Chinese, Mexican, Italian, and Jewish diets plus meals for camping, traveling, holidays, school lunches, children's parties, and many other special occasions. It's an essential handbook for all who want varied, exciting, and flexible dining.

Although we have all of these books at the Sugarfree Center, you ought to be able to find them at your own local bookstore. If you can't, you ought to yell at them until they stock them because they are books that should be readily available.

Now, while we don't feel it's necessary for us to reinvent the wheel of diabetic recipes and exchanges here, we'd yell at ourselves if we neglected to pass on a few of our favorite dining and cooking tips that we feel help make life a little easier, healthier, or more fun.

GROW HERBS

Herbs are almost as easy to grow as weeds (which some, such as mint, practically are). You can fill up corners of the yard with them, or you can put them in pots in a window if you live in an apartment. The difference they make in the taste of food is amazing. Just a few fresh herbs cut up in a salad move it into the realm of the ambrosial. (Tip: Chop up a couple of mint leaves along with the other herbs. It gives a fresh taste but not a decidedly minty one.)

Grow oregano. Grow dill. Grow rosemary. Grow coriander (great in Oriental and Mexican dishes). Grow sage. Grow marjoram. Grow tarragon—if you can. It's one of Barbara's favorites, but she's had bad luck trying to get a good crop of it. Basil, on the other hand, always flourishes. Basil takes us back to the two times we've been allowed to stay at a friend's house in a small town in Provence. Pots of it are sold in the market, and you can keep it on your kitchen sink and snip away, putting bits of it in practically everything. Add it and garlic to your favorite vegetable soup and voilà, you have *soupe au pistou*. Basil is also invaluable if you follow our next admonition.

EAT PASTA

If you want to check out the findings of the Glycemic Index (see chapter 14), try adding a lot more pasta to your diet. You may find, as June does, that it's the least damaging starch, blood-sugarily speaking. Don't think of it as fattening. It's not, especially if you keep the fat down in sauces. Try this recipe with some of your fresh basil. It's a modification of one Nora Ephron had in her novel *Heartburn*. Yes, novel. You should read it. Not only do you get all the backstairs gossip of the breakup of her marriage to Carl Bernstein (of Woodward and Bernstein fame), but you get fifteen dandy recipes as well.

Pasta alla Cecca

Drop 5 large tomatoes in boiling water for 1 full minute. Peel and seed and chop. Put in a large bowl with 2 tablespoons of olive oil, a garlic clove sliced in two, 1 cup chopped fresh basil leaves, as little salt as possible (or even none), and as many red hot pepper flakes as you feel up to. Let this sit for a couple of hours, then remove the garlic. (If you really like garlic, chop it or press it and leave it in.) Boil 1 pound of pasta (linguine, spaghetti, or what you will). Serve immediately. As Nora Ephron says, "It's a hot pasta with a cold tomato and basil sauce, and it's so light and delicate that it's almost like eating a salad." If you divide the sauce into 8 servings, each will be 1 vegetable exchange and a trace of a fat exchange (the best kind!). Pasta is 1 bread exchange per half cup.

(Later on, if you find pasta works as well for you as it does for June, you could alow yourself a little extra.)

Pasta can carry off all kinds of sauces. Investigate recipes in the above cookbooks; experiment on your own. For store-bought dry pasta we recommend getting the imported variety. It's much superior. Good brands are Agnesi and De Cecco, and the best of all is Martelli. Or you could make your own. It's not all that difficult if you have a pasta maker (get the hand-crank model—for home use you don't need the electric one). Barbara used to make pasta a lot although she had problems with her cat knocking all the pasta off the drying rack and onto the floor in a heap. Thus was born a new dish: Pasta alla Mishka. A combination of linguine and spaghetti and lasagne noodles all mixed up and broken up. But she doesn't make pasta much anymore because she follows the advice to . . .

GET BY WITH A LITTLE HELP
FROM YOUR FRIENDS

Another wonderful trend in this country is the rise of little ethnic delicatessens where you can purchase dishes to take home for dinner. French housewives have been doing this for years. Now American men and women who have less and less time to cook are availing themselves of the offerings of these new establishments. You do have to check them out, though, to make sure they do your kind of cooking; that is, low in fat and sugar and salt.

Just when our time was in shortest supply and we needed it most, an Italian delicatessen opened only about two miles away. Zio's (meaning "Uncle's") it's called, and it makes all kinds of home-made pastas and soups and salads, and it makes them our way. Here's a sample recipe:

Minestrone allo Zio

1½ cups dried cannellini beans (white kidney beans)
8 ounces fresh spinach
2 celery ribs
2 carrots

1 large potato
2 small zucchini
1 small bunch Swiss chard
1 small head savoy cabbage (wrinkled type)
¼ cup chopped Italian parsley
2 garlic cloves (chopped)
2 tablespoons olive oil
1 medium red onion
2 quarts (approximately) of chicken or meat broth

Soak beans in 3 cups of cold water overnight. Drain and cook beans for 40 minutes in lightly salted water.

Wash Swiss chard, spinach, and cabbage, then cut into strips and, with only the water left on the leaves after washing, cook in another saucepan for 20 minutes. Drain excess water from cooked vegetables and set aside.

Place parsley, garlic, and olive oil in a stockpot, and saute gently for 15 minutes.

Cut celery, carrot, potato, zucchini, and onion into small (¼ to ½ inch) pieces. Add to stockpot, and saute with the garlic and parsley for an additional 5 minutes.

Transfer the partially cooked beans and 1 cup of their water to the stockpot, then add the spinach mixture.

Add broth (enough to cover the vegetables by approximately 4 inches), and simmer slowly until all vegetables are cooked (about 1 hour).

If you divide this into 10 servings, each one will be 2 vegetable exchanges, ½ bread, and ½ fat.

Of course, many times you won't feel like cooking, and you won't even feel like bringing food in, you'll want to *go out*, and in that case . . .

DON'T FORGET THE DOGGIE BAG

With the exception of some of those more extreme *cuisine min-ceur* establishments, almost all restaurants serve twice as much food as you need. For that reason the doggie bag has become *de rigueur* in even V.E.F.Rs. and V.E.I.Rs. Some even present your leavings and takings in artistic foil swans. Naturally if you were dining out with Prince Charles and Lady Di you probably wouldn't want to ask for a doggie bag, but under almost any other circumstances it's okay. It's lovely to have the food the next day. It's even lovelier to know you didn't overdo the night before. To prevent this overdoing, we heard an interesting tip. Ask for your doggie bag at the *beginning* of the meal. Leave on your plate only what is on your diet for that meal, and put the rest in the doggie bag to avoid temptation and an absent-minded eating-too-much. It's a good habit to get into, and you should always try to . . .

ESTABLISH GOOD HABITS

We have an acquaintance who says with pride, "In our house Friday night is martini and hamburger night." This means, we later found out, that she and her husband always celebrate the end of the week by zonking themselves on martinis and then gorging themselves on hamburgers. Habitually. It's just as easy to establish good habits and learn to cherish them. At the Sugarfree Center we always celebrate the end of the week by having:

Always on Friday Bran Muffins
(a modification of a *Laurel's Kitchen* recipe)

1 cup whole wheat flour
1 teaspoon baking soda
½ teaspoon Life Salt (or light salt)
2 tablespoons fructose
1 cup Quaker Oat Bran Cereal
½ cup wheat bran
2 tablespoons oil
2 tablespoons molasses
1½ cups buttermilk
1 egg
1/3 cup chopped walnuts

Preheat oven to 375 F. Mix dry ingredients together. Combine oil and molasses; add beaten egg and buttermilk. Add liquid to dry ingredients, and stir until moistened. Stir in nuts.

Fill Pam-sprayed muffin tins 2/3 full, and bake 20 minutes. Makes 13 muffins. Each equals 1 bread and 1 fat exchange.

But you don't have to take on our good habits, you can think up your own if you . . .

USE YOUR IMAGINATION

Now is the time to break out of your old eating patterns. Try something you've never tried before out of the diabetic cookbooks. Then when you're feeling more venturesome go out to a kind of restaurant you've never been to and try a dish you've never tasted. Try sushi, those delectable little rice cylinders with a delicate piece of raw fish on top. Note: June says you don't *have* to try sushi. Okay, if the raw fish is too much for you try something different. Try couscous. If you don't have a restaurant serving couscous in your hometown (we lucky devils in Los Angeles have three of them), you can make it at home.

Couscous

Take 4 cups of cracked wheat, and soak it in approximately 2 cups of cold water for 1 hour. Occasionally run your fingers through it to break up lumps.

There is such a thing as a special couscous cooker, but we don't have one so we use a steaming pot that's kind of like a double boiler with holes in the top section. You can also use a large pot with a collander set in it. In the bottom section of whatever you're using put about 1½ pounds of lean beef or lamb or chicken cut in 1½-inch cubes. Add 2 thinly sliced onions, 1 teaspoon of grated fresh ginger (or ½ teaspoon of ground ginger), freshly ground pepper to taste, 3 cloves, 1 teaspoon turmeric, ¼ teaspoon nutmeg, and 2 tablespoons butter or oil. Cook the meat just up to the point of browning; then add water or chicken broth so it comes up to about 2 inches above the other ingredients.

Place the collander (or whatever you're using) in the pot, and bring the pot to a boil.

Line the collander with cheesecloth, and add the couscous—again breaking up any lumps that may have formed. Cover and simmer for about 45 minutes, letting the couscous steam.

Remove the collander, and set it aside. Put into the pot 3 carrots cut in quarters, 4 turnips peeled and quartered, 3 medium zucchini cut into 1-inch pieces, 2 medium-small onions quartered, and ¼ cup seedless raisins. (Classic couscous also calls for garbanzos, but we usually leave them out, figuring it's better to concentrate your major carbohydrate on the wheat). When these have almost cooked to the degree of doneness you like, put the couscous back on top again to reheat.

To serve, put the couscous on a platter and arrange the meat and vegetables on top. Garnish with almonds. Accompany it with a bowl of sauce from the pot and a dish of hot sauce. (We use a Mexican one because it's easy to find in the stores.)

Guests can be given bowls into which they can put the couscous and meat and vegetables along with a little broth and hot sauce if they like. Ideally they should eat it with their hands (their right hands only) while reclining on pillows on the floor. Of course, as a good host or hostess you'll have already washed their hands for them with water that has rose petals floating in it.

Since everything is so identifiable, if you keep in mind that the cracked wheat is 1 bread exchange for each 1/3 cup, you should have no trouble calculating the rest of your meal.

For dessert, although it's a bit out of the appropriate region, we suggest a spiced tea we were served in a spice garden near Matale in Sri Lanka. It was delicious, but it tasted so sweet that we kept asking the guide if he was certain it had no sugar in it. To prove it didn't he gave us the recipe.

Sri Lankan Spiced Tea

Bring 4 cups of water to a boil in a pan. Add 2 teaspoons of tea, a piece of ginger, a piece of cinnamon, 1 mace flower, and 2 cardamom seeds. Boil together for 15 minutes. Stir, and add 3 or 4 drops of vanilla.

CARBOHYDRATE AND CALORIC VALUES OF ALCOHOLIC BEVERAGES

Ida Jaqua

Beverage	Amount	Calories	Grams of Carbo- hydrate
Ale, Beer			
Ale, domestic	8 ounces	104	8
Beer, domestic	8 ounces	114	10⅜
Champale	8 ounces	127	10
Cocktails, Premixed			
Black Velvet (Heublein)	1 ounce	65	0
Daiquiri (Calvert)	1 ounce	63	3
Daiquiri (Heublein)	1 ounce	59	4
Daiquiri (Hiram Walker)	1 ounce	59	4
Manhattan (Calvert)	1 ounce	54	¾
Manhattan (Hiram Walker)	1 ounce	49	1
Margarita (Calvert)	1 ounce	59	3
Margarita (Heublein)	1 ounce	48	2
Martini (Calvert)	1 ounce	59	0
Martini (Heublein)	1 ounce	56	⅜
Martini (Hiram Walker)	1 ounce	56	¼
Old Fashioned (Hiram Walker)	1 ounce	55	1

Beverage	Amount	Calories	Grams of Carbo- hydrate
Vodka martini (Hiram Walker)	1 ounce	49	0
Whiskey sour (Calvert)	1 ounce	65	3
Whiskey sour (Hiram Walker)	1 ounce	59	4

Distilled Spirits*

80 proof	1 ounce	67	0
84 proof	1 ounce	70	0
86 proof	1 ounce	72	0
90 proof	1 ounce	75	0
94 proof	1 ounce	78	0
94.6 proof	1 ounce	79	0
97 proof	1 ounce	81	0
100 proof	1 ounce	83	0

Liqueurs, Cordials

Akvavit (Aalborg Regular)	1 ounce	62	⅛
Akvavit (Aalborg Jubilaeums)	1 ounce	62	2½
Anisette (Bols)	1 ounce	111	14
Anisette (Hiram Walker)	1 ounce	92	10¾
Apricot cordial (Hiram Walker)	1 ounce	82	8⅓
Apricot-flavored brandy (Hiram Walker)	1 ounce	88	7½
Blackberry brandy (Bols)	1 ounce	100	7⅗

* Bourbon, brandy, cognac, Canadian whiskey, gin, rye, rum, scotch, tequila, vodka.

Beverage	Amount	Calories	Grams of Carbo- hydrate
Liqueurs, Cordials (*cont.*)			
Blackberry cordial (Hiram Walker)	1 ounce	100	12¾
Blackberry-flavored brandy (Hiram Walker)	1 ounce	86	7
Blackberry liqueur (Bols)	1 ounce	96	9
Cherry cordial (Hiram Walker)	1 ounce	82	8
Cherry heering (Hiram Walker)	1 ounce	80	10
Coffee southern (Southern Comfort)	1 ounce	85	7
Crème de Cacao (Bols)	1 ounce	101	11⅘
Crème de Cacao (Hiram Walker regular or white)	1 ounce	104	15
Crème de Menthe (Bols)	1 ounce	112	13
Crème de Menthe (Hiram Walker green or white)	1 ounce	94	11⅕
Crème de Noyaux (Bols)	1 ounce	115	13¾
Curacao (Bols blue)	1 ounce	105	10⅓
Curacao (Bols orange)	1 ounce	100	8⅘
Curacao (Hiram Walker orange)	1 ounce	96	11¾
Drambuie (Hiram Walker)	1 ounce	110	11
Ginger-flavored brandy (Hiram Walker)	1 ounce	72	3½

Beverage	*Amount*	*Calories*	*Grams of Carbo-hydrate*
Irish Mist	1 ounce	120	5⅗
Kümmel (Hiram Walker)	1 ounce	71	3¾
Peach cordial (Hiram Walker)	1 ounce	81	8
Peach-flavored brandy (Hiram Walker)	1 ounce	87	7⅕
Peppermint schnapps (Hiram Walker)	1 ounce	78	7⅕
Rock and rye (Hiram Walker)	1 ounce	87	9½
Sloe gin (Bols)	1 ounce	85	4¾
Sloe gin (Hiram Walker)	1 ounce	68	4¾
Southern Comfort	1 ounce	120	3½
Tia Maria (Hiram Walker)	1 ounce	92	10
Triple sec (Bols)	1 ounce	113	8⅘
Triple sec (Hiram Walker)	1 ounce	105	9¾

Wines

Champagne, brut	3 ounces	75	1
Champagne, extra dry	3 ounces	87	3¾
Dubonnet (Schenley)	3 ounces	96	7
Marsala (Florio dry)	3 ounces	162	18
Marsala (Florio sweet)	3 ounces	182	23
Mirin (Kiku-Masamure)	3 ounces	225	36
Port, Ruby	3 ounces	138	10
Port, Tawny	3 ounces	138	11
Red table wine (dry)	3 ounces	69	trace

Beverage	*Amount*	*Calories*	*Grams of Carbo-hydrate*
Wines (*cont.*)			
Sake (Kiku-Masamure)	3 ounces	75	6
Sherry, dry	3 ounces	120	1
Sherry, sweet	3 ounces	150	6
Vermouth, dry	3½ ounces	105	1
Vermouth, sweet	3½ ounces	167	12
White table wine (dry)	3 ounces	74	trace
Mixers, Soft Drinks			
Bitter lemon (Schweppes)	10 ounces	160	39⅖
Bitter orange (Schweppes)	10 ounces	153	37¾
Catawba sparkling grape juice	3 ounces	58	14¾
Club soda (Schweppes)	10 ounces	0	0
Ginger ale (Schweppes)	10 ounces	110	27
Ginger beer (Schweppes)	10 ounces	120	29⅖
Lime juice (Rose's sweetened)	1 ounce	49	12
Moxie	10 ounces	129	29
Tonic water (Schweppes)	10 ounces	110	27½

METER READER: THE SUGARFREE CENTER UNSCIENTIFIC AND OPINIONATED REPORT ON METERS

At the moment there are six blood-sugar testing meters on the market. By the time you read this there may be seven or eight or nine, or some that we already have may have come out in new, improved models. Manufacturer competition and meter technology are advancing at a dizzying pace. Meters are becoming more accurate, simpler to operate, and lower in price. And more and more insurance firms are picking up a percentage of the tab. Now even Medicare is paying for meters and supplies for insulin-dependent diabetics who have frequent insulin reactions, hyperglycemia, and ketosis. (In a sense, they reward you for being out of control.)

Many of you use visually read strips to keep track of your blood sugar—either Chemstrips bG or Visidex II strips. This is the inexpensive way to go and can work well for noninsulin-dependent diabetics with good vision and color judgment. For the insulin-dependent, for pregnant women, for the extremely brittle, getting a ball-park figure by eye is often not precise enough for good therapy. If you learn to be a careful operator, a meter can give you much more laboratorylike blood-sugar readings.

The leading question of most diabetics who come to the Sugarfree Center to select a meter is, "Which one is the most accurate?" (Even a twelve-year-old boy asked this question first after a demonstration of all the meters.) We have searched in vain for an unbiased scientific study comparing results from all the different meters. No such comprehensive study exists.

It's true that almost every manufacturer will be able to provide you with a study—usually done at a university or hospital—that proves its meter to be the most accurate. Cynics that we are, we have the feeling that when the manufacturer gives the financial backing to the study, the scientific cards may be stacked in such a way that its meter tends to come out on top. If it doesn't, the study is not likely to be published and distributed by the manufacturer. (No fools they!)

Neither have we been able to get firsthand scientific evaluations of meters from nurses, hospital laboratories, or physicians' offices. Their feedback is conflicting. We have often loaned different brands of meters to hospital staffs so that they could compare results of portable meters with hospital laboratory results and select one for nursing staff use. One hospital will choose a certain meter with unqualified enthusiasm and reject another as giving poor results on their comparison tests. A different hospital will conduct its own tests and come back wanting to purchase the very meter rejected by the first hospital. (We suspect that the variations in meter accuracy are often not the fault of the meter but are in reality variations in the strips. Our suspicions were confirmed in experiments performed by diabetic lab technician Dixie Starkovitch.) At any rate, since the professionals do not agree among themselves, we are left with a great befuddlement.

To help diabetics sort out the advantages and disadvantages of the different meters and make a wise personal choice, we have prepared this "Sugarfree Center Unscientific and Opinionated Report on Meters." Our report is unscientific because it is not based on tests performed in a laboratory on rats. It is based on what scientists like to dismiss as "anecdotal evidence." Our definition of *anecdotal evidence* is "what really happens to real people and they tell you about it." In the following analysis of meters we'll tell you what we have learned during the past three years by using meters ourselves, by teaching their use to hundreds of diabetics, and by receiving comments from letter writers who have shared with us their enthusiasms and disgruntlements with meters.

As a general preliminary statement, we can say that all the meters on the market are accurate within 10 percent (plus or minus). They can also be inaccurate if you, the operator, use sloppy techniques or do not keep your meter clean and well serviced according to the manufacturer's instructions. All of the meters perform the same function—after you apply a drop of blood from your fingertip to the testing strip and remove the blood at the specified time by washing, wiping, or blotting, you put the strip into the meter and it gives you a digital readout of your blood-sugar level. So when you choose a meter, you are also choosing a strip. First, then, we must consider the types of strips.

STRIPS USED IN METERS

There are at present three strips used in meters—Dextrostix, Chemstrips bG, and Glucoscan strips. Some meters can read one brand of strip only. Other meters have models to read more than one type of strip. Many people prefer to have a meter that uses Chemstrips bG because they then have what the engineers call "the redundancy factor." You can read the strip visually as well as in the meter, so you'll be able to see if there is a wide discrepancy between the two, which might indicate a meter (or operator!) malfunction.

Here are the characteristics of the different strips.

Dextrostix

Availability: most pharmacies
Packaging: 25s and 100s (in a glass container)
Cost each at Sugarfree Center: $.42
Size of pad:

Timing of test: 1 minute
Blood removal: wash with water and blot
Visual reading: difficult, not recommended
Stability: must be read immediately, not stable

Chemstrips bG

Availability: most pharmacies
Packaging: 25s and 50s (in a metal container)
Cost each at Sugarfree Center: $.45
Size of pad:

Timing of test: 2 minutes
Blood removal: wipe with tissue or cotton
Visual reading: easy; strip is designed for visual reading
Stability: 7 days in an airtight container

Glucoscan Test Strips

Availability· from Lifescan (manufacturer) by mail and a few distributors such as the Sugarfree Center
Packaging: 50s and 100s (individually wrapped in foil)
Cost each at Sugarfree Center: $.44
Size of pad:

Timing of test: 1 minute
Blood removal: blot on special paper supplied with strips
Visual reading: difficult, not recommended
Stability: must be read immediately, not stable

METERS
METERS FOR DEXTROSTIX

Glucometer

Manufactured by the Ames Division, Miles Laboratories, Inc. (P.O. Box 70, Elkhart, IN 46515; 219-264-8284). Made in U.S.A. It came on the market in 1981 as the first battery-operated small home-use meter and originally sold for $250. Available through Ames Self-Testing Centers.

Dimensions: 3.25″ by 6.60″ by 1.3″
Weight: 12 ounces (including batteries)
Power supply: 4 AA batteries
Shut off: manual
Timing of test: 1 minute
Reading range: 0–400 mg/dl
Price: $150
Guarantee: 1 year

The Glucometer can be purchased only in an approved Ames

Self-Testing Center, as a one-hour training session is necessary. It requires considerable sophistication to operate, as the user must calibrate it each time a new bottle of strips is opened and must run a control test. This means that three Dextrostix are used up before you even take your first blood sugar. The Glucometer can also be calibrated with the two calibration chips provided with the meter, but that makes for less accuracy.

Below the display panel there is an on/off switch and three buttons (Calibrate, Read, and Time). This can be confusing during low blood-sugar states or the early morning groggies.

This is a reliable, tried and true machine but now somewhat outmoded in technology. And few people like a wash strip.

BetaScan A

Distributed by Orange Medical Instruments (3183 Airway Avenue, Suite F, Costa Mesa, CA 92626; 213-614-5836). Made in England. Sold by Diabetes Education Centers and some distributors such as the Sugarfree Center.

Dimensions: 3.9″ by 6.7″ by 1.2″
Weight: 10 ounces
Power supply: built-in rechargeable batteries
Shut off: manual
Timing of test: 1 minute
Reading range: 0–400 mg/dl
Price: $250
Guarantee: 1 year

The BetaScan A is self-calibrating. A fresh Dextrostix is inserted into the meter before each test to set calibration. The meter takes nine seconds for the calibration. When you remove the strip you have eight seconds to apply a drop of blood before automatic timing begins. The LED readout is red and particularly easy to read. The machine has an excessively loud buzzer.

The BetaScan A is an improvement over the Glucometer in that it is self-calibrating and has only two control buttons (On/Off and Test), but it must be recharged for twenty-four hours each week. This is something of a nuisance to most people.

METERS FOR CHEMSTRIPS bG

Accu-Chek bG

The makers of Chemstrips bG, Bio-Dynamics (9115 Hague Road, Indianapolis, IN 46250; 317-845-2000), market this meter. Made in Germany. Sold through Bio-Dynamics Diabetes Supply Centers; a lesson is necessary at time of purchase. The original price was $265.

Dimensions: 3.5″ by 7.1″ by 1.5″
Weight: 14 ounces (with batteries)
Power supply: 4 AA alkaline batteries
Shut off: automatic after 5 minutes
Timing of test: 2 minutes
Reading range: 40–400 mg/dl
Price: $150
Guarantee: 1 year

The Accu-Chek bG can only be used with Chemstrips bG in packages of fifty, as these contain a special calibration filmstrip that must be inserted in the meter and left there as long as the package of Chemstrips is in use. (The calibration strip and the vial of Chemstrips must have the same lot number.) This special calibration system, which enhances accuracy, is a feature that makes the meter popular with hospitals and doctors' offices.

An unused Chemstrip must be placed in the meter and the test-strip door closed and opened before you can take your test. This door, which is rather large and awkward, must be opened and closed twice for each test.

The aperture window through which the meter reads the strip is right on top and is exposed when the door is open. If the window is not kept extremely clean, the meter will refuse to calibrate. Occasionally it is temperamental and refuses to function if you close the door in a jerky, unsmooth manner. The nine messages it gives you on the display are a little cryptic (for example, ELO equals Calibration Strip Error, and PPP equals Low Batteries). But these are small prices to pay for the accuracy for which this meter is known.

Glucochek II

Imported by Larken Industries, Ltd. (8397 Melrose, Lenexa, KS 66214; 1-800-452-7536). Made in England. Available from a small network of highly selected distributors, including the Sugar-free Center.

Dimensions: 6.6" by 2.9" by .95"
Weight: 9 ounces (including batteries)
Power supply: 4 AA alkaline batteries
Shut off: automatic after 3 minutes
Timing of test: 2 minutes
Reading range: 10–400 mg/dl
Price: $250
Guarantee: 1 year

No buttons to push, only a small door to open and close. Automatic calibration is performed by inserting an unused strip. The display immediately reads Go, if the strip is okay. When your drop of blood is ready, remove the strip. You have five seconds to apply the blood before automatic timing starts. Buzzer warns at sixty seconds for wiping the strip and at zero for reading it. Insert the strip and close the door for your blood-sugar reading. Definitely the most automatic of the meters. The only caution is that you have to be fast enough to get your blood on the strip in the five seconds allotted. Favored by hospital neonatal (newborn) units because of its ability to read down to 10 mg/dl.

A marvelous plus for the Glucochek II is that you can purchase a strip cutter and a half strip track to use with the meter. The cost to convert to half strips is $29.95. Using the half strip method means the price of each test is only twenty-two cents and you need half as much blood as with a full strip. Half strips are also easier to cover fully and this ensures more accuracy.

There is an alternate model of the Glucochek II that reads Dextrostix.

Glucokey

Imported from England by Ulster Scientific, Inc. (P.O. Box 902, Highland, NY 12528; 1-800-431-8232), the people who brought you the Autolet. The meter is sold only as a system with an Autolet, a battery charger, and a carrying case. Available from selected distributors.

Dimensions: 5" by 4.5" by 1.7"
Weight: 13 ounces
Power supply: electric current and rechargeable batteries (included)
Shut off: automatic after 3 minutes
Timing of test: 2 minutes
Reading range: 18–360 mg/dl
Price: $229
Guarantee: 1 year

This meter is made of bright blue plastic and opens with a not-unobtrusive grinding sound. Two buttons—Timer and Test. The calibration process is a dual operation of inserting a fresh strip and after that a special standard strip (only one is supplied with the meter). To complete a test you must push buttons five times: On, Calibrate 1, Calibrate 2, Time (sixty seconds), Time (sixty seconds more), and Test. As each step is completed the meter sounds a three-note tone, causing some wags to nickname it the "music box."

To use the meter on batteries you must recharge it for fourteen hours whenever they get low.

The Glucokey is available in an alternate version (A), which reads Dextrostix, and a third version (C), which reads Key Reagent Strips. Though Key strips have been announced they were not yet available when this report was compiled.

METERS FOR GLUCOSCAN TEST STRIPS

Glucoscan II

This meter is manufactured by Lifescan, Inc. (1025 Terra Bella Avenue, Mountain View, CA 94043; 1-800-227-8862, in California 1-800-982-6132) in northern California's famous Silicon Valley. The meter and strips are available directly from Lifescan or from selected distributors, including the Sugarfree Center. The original price of the Glucoscan II was $219.

Dimensions: 5.5″ by 3.2″ by .57″
Weight: 6 ounces (with battery)
Power supply: J battery
Shut off: automatic after 3 minutes
Timing of test: 1 minute
Reading range: 40–450 mg/dl
Price: $159
Guarantee: 1 year

The smallest, fastest, and most portable meter. Factory calibrated. Three buttons—On, Time, and Test. Glucoscan Test Strips are individual foil-wrapped strips with small pads. They are blotted at the end of forty seconds on the special blotting paper supplied with them. A discreet sound signals you to read the strip at the end of the minute.

Precisely timed blotting technique is essential for accuracy. And one other word of caution: With blood sugars over 450 the Glucoscan II may read out any figure up to 900, but these are not correct and *under no circumstances should you base your insulin dosage on these false high figures*.

Lifescan's Customer Service, available on their 800 number, is especially accommodating and helpful.

METER POPULARITY CONTEST

Each of the meters has its passionate advocates who claim that it is the most accurate, the easiest to use, the most reliable, and the most clever. And each has doctors, nurses, and diabetics who reject these same meters, claiming, "It's no good," "It's not working," "It doesn't match the lab result," and other such condemnations.

In our experience *all* the meters work well, but, as we said before, not without good technique and good care. We have witnessed even professionals trying to get accurate blood sugars with the most inept of performances—not enough blood on the strip, too much time used applying the blood, blood applied unevenly, blood scrubbed onto the strip instead of being allowed to flow on, timer button pushed too late, blood not fully wiped off, pad wiped too vigorously, strip placed in the meter backward or not completely inserted.

We have taken trade-in Glucometers that were so filthy they must have been giving the most fanciful of blood sugars. We cannot preach too strongly that meters are scientific instruments that must be handled with precision and serviced· regularly.

Different meters appeal to different people and for different reasons. All the meters have plusses and minuses. You have to select your own meter with the advice and counsel of your physician and/ or nurse educator. Buying a meter is like buying a house or a car or even like falling in love. Your personality and lifestyle and emotions are often the deciding factors in your choice. Therefore, we can't tell you which meter you should get. We can, however, tell you how the meters have done on the Sugarfree Center Billfold Ballot, that is to say which ones our clients are currently buying.

> In early 1983, the Glucoscan II outsold all other meters and is still selling well.
> In late 1983, the Glucochek II has moved out in front in spite of not lowering its price. The strip-cutting feature may be responsible in part for this increase in sales.
> The Accu-Chek is gaining since the firm lowered its price and since the meter became more readily available.
> The Glucometer is hardly selling at all.
> The BetaScan has been selected by only one person and that was because it was the meter prescribed by the doctor. Three have been sold to be shipped to an Air Force hospital in Greece.
> We did not offer the Glucokey at the time this survey was taken.

As changes take place on the meter scene, we'll continually update this report in future issues of the Sugarfree Center *Health-O-Gram* (write for a free copy and subscription information: P.O. Box 114, Van Nuys, CA 91408.)

IN AN EMERGENCY

Even the most fit business travelers are, from time to time, faced with illness or accidents when they are away from home; and at the same time, people with medical problems frequently must travel on business.

In recent years, a number of medical aids, organizations, and other services have been developed to help those in need cope with emergencies. Each serves slightly different situations.

One group deals with the paraphernalia—bracelets, necklaces, tags, cards—that identifies the wearer's health problem and other pertinent information and enables a medic, hospital, or doctor to have or to obtain a patient's medical history quickly.

MediScope, Microdesign Systems/BS, 101 Fifth Avenue, New York, NY 10003. MediScope is a pendant, smaller than a thimble and worn on a necklace, that contains one's name, address, phone, and medical record on microfilm that can be read immediately by the simple device of a minuscule built-in magnifying glass. To view the information, an emergency attendant need only hold the pendant to a light.

The device could save the life of someone with heart trouble, diabetes, or another serious condition when time is of the essence, since the essential information is immediately available. Cost is $14.95, and information can be updated for $3.

Medic Alert, Medic Alert Foundation, P.O. Box 1009, Turlock, CA 95381. The stainless steel Medic Alert emblem, which can be worn as a bracelet or necklace, is engraved on the back with the wearer's medical problem and an I.D. number and phone number that can be called twenty-four hours a day collect from anywhere in the world. In addition to the emblem, members carry a wallet-size computer printout of their file that provides personal and medical information.

The emergency answering service can retrieve the person's medical history, family data, and other vital and appropriate information stored in a member's file. A one-time charge for life membership is $15. Medic Alert has affiliates in sixteen countries.

Medical DataCard, U.S. Medicom Corporation, 65 South 21st Street, Kenilworth, NJ 07033. Medical DataCard is a plastic card containing pertinent health and personal information. The most urgent information is visible to the naked eye; other data can be read with a doctor's ophthalmoscope. Cost is $19, and updates are $8. The company is arranging to have computer access to the information through an emergency 800 number.

Medical Data Banc, Medical Data Banc Inc., 7920 Ward Parkway, Kansas City, MO 64114. A plastic credit card–size identification card has the full medical history of the holder and optional authorization for specific treatments and surgery. The laminated card carries the data on microfilm that can be read on any standard microfilm reader. Cost is $18 individual, $36 family for a three-year subscription.

If a reader is not available, the card bears a toll-free number that can be called from anywhere in the world. It is answered on a twenty-four-hour basis at the computer center in Kansas City, where operators read the needed information to the caller.

In addition to optional authorizations for treatment and the holder's name, address, and description, the card includes such information as the employer's name, insurance company, type of insurance, personal physician, persons to notify in case of emergency, special instructions, religion, blood type, previous illness, etc.

A second group of organizations is designed to provide a range of emergency medical and related assistance to travelers, particularly in unfamiliar surroundings.

MediCall International, Three Landmark Sq., Stamford, CT 06901. A subsidiary of Credit Card Service Corporation of Alexandria, Virginia, the membership/insurance organization provides medical assistance services in case of injury or illness for members traveling 100 miles from home in the United States or abroad. The MediCall International Response Center, its emergency communications system, operates twenty-four hours a day, 365 days a year and can be reached by telephone or telex.

Its long list of available services—depending on the program selected—includes telephone referral to appropriate medical facilities; emergency medical transportation; round-trip transportation for one friend or relative to join a disabled member confined to a hospital bed for seven days or more who was traveling alone; return of unattended minors to member's home, accompanied when required; medically equipped emergency aircraft in key locations; ambulances for evacuation services and to move a member to hospital or clinic.

Membership is available to individuals as well as to companies on a per trip or annual basis. The most comprehensive program costs $75 for individuals and $90 for a family per year or $25 and $40 for a single trip for up to thirty days.

There are several corporate programs available, and they cover field offices as well as headquarters locations. Programs can be purchased directly from the company or through travel agents.

Health Care Abroad, International Underwriters/Brokers, Inc., 1029 Investment Building, 1511 K Street N.W., Washington, DC 20005. The health insurance package for $2 a day provides a range of emergency transportation and medical services, major medical insurance, and accident and sickness benefits with a minimum premium of $25.

Members receive a directory of participating physicians and hospitals worldwide and twenty-four-hour telephone referral service and membership card to be used in lieu of payment after a $50 deductible.

A third group is designed to provide medical information on countries around the world, lists of English-speaking doctors, and pretravel counseling.

IAMAT, International Association for Medical Assistance to Travelers, 736 Center Street, Lewiston, NY 14092. IAMAT is a nonprofit organization whose membership and publications are free of charge, although a donation is requested.

In addition to its directory of doctors, it publishes a variety of booklets on world climate, immunization, and medical conditions, and has made itself something of a worldwide health watchdog issuing health alerts on areas having high-risk potential. IAMAT will respond to written requests for information on a specific location and needs up to five weeks to respond.

Intermedic, 777 Third Avenue, New York, NY 10017. The organization provides medical information and doctor lists for countries around the world and has a personal medical data form to be completed by the member's physician for use when visiting a doctor elsewhere in the world. Membership is $6 for individuals, $10 for a family per year.

International Health Care Service, The New York Hospital–Cornell Medical Center, 525 East 68th Street, New York, NY 10021. The center offers seminars, booklets, pretravel counseling, and immunizations on a per fee basis. It has a posttravel diagnostic procedure, disease treatment, emergency medical facilities, and worldwide physician information system. The service also offers corporate health programs. Prices range from $8–$15 for immunizations and $50–$100 for travel health plans.

A fourth group of organizations assists travelers with a wide range of emergency situations in addition to health and medical ones.

Assist-Card, Assist-Card Corporation of America, 745 Fifth Avenue, New York, NY 10022. Assist-Card is a traveler's emergency assistance organization to provide help in fifty-six countries. It is staffed twenty-four hours a day with multilingual service representatives who provide members free qualified doctors and hospitalization for unexpected illness or accident costing up to $3,000; emergency contact to member's home; legal assistance for accident-related problems, and a loan of up to $5,000 to meet bail requirements; lost travel documents and tickets retrieval or replacement; and other emergency help.

Cost of Assist-Card is based on the number of days of travel abroad and is approximately $3 per day. The card can be purchased through travel agents or directly from the company.

International SOS Assistance, Philadelphia Executive Offices,

Two Neshaminy Interplex, Trevose, PA 19047. The membership organization in cooperation with International Service Corporation, a subsidiary of INA Corporation of Philadelphia, offers medical and nonmedical emergency assistance for travelers, such as legal assistance, interpreters, and cash advances. Medical assistance includes emergency evacuation of an injured member as well as flying family members to the bedside of a sick or injured person, among other benefits. Membership is available on an individual, short-term basis of $12.50 for seven days or annually. There are also group and corporations subscriptions as well as special arrangements for Avis President's Club members.

Additionally, there are organizations whose main function is emergency evacuation in case of illness or accident.

AIR-EVAC, Air-Evac International, Inc., 296 "H" Street, Suite 301, Chula Vista, CA 92010. The company is specialized in air medical evacuation of emergency patients from foreign countries back to the United States. It uses medically staffed and outfitted aircraft and has an air-to-ground communications system. Fees are based on service; the basic program starts at $25 for individuals per year for up to $10,000 of services and $35 for a family for up to $30,000. For travel farther than 1,500 miles from the United States, a higher rate scale pertains. Foreign hospitalization insurance is also available through the program.

NEAR, Nationwide/Worldwide Emergency Ambulance Return, 1900 North MacArthur Blvd., Suite 210, Oklahoma City, OK 73127. For $120 a year per person (or $2 per day) the organization provides emergency air and ground transportation to a member's home from anywhere in the world in case of illness, injury, or death.

Finally, there are special arrangements made by travel companies for their clients. For example, **Hertz** customers traveling in ten European countries, who take personal accident insurance when renting a Hertz car, receive free emergency medical treatment and hospitalization, if needed, through an arrangement with Europ Assistance.

When necessary, the service includes free transportation by air ambulance, accompanied by medical staff, to a hospital or clinic in the United States, a friend to travel with the disabled person or free round-trip ticket for family member, if patient is unable to travel.

MEMBER ASSOCIATIONS OF THE INTERNATIONAL DIABETES FEDERATION

EUROPEAN REGION

AUSTRIA

OSTERREICHISCHER DIABETIKERVERBAND,
Pfeilgasse 43, A-1080 VIENNA.

OSTERREICHISCHE DIABETESGESELLSCHAFT,
c/o Dr. G. Schernthaner (Secretary), Department of Medicine II, University of Vienna, Garnisongasse 13, A-1090 VIENNA.

BELGIUM

ASSOCIATION BELGE DU DIABETE,
234b Avenue Winston Churchill, B-1180 BRUXELLES.
Telephone (02) 344 06 95.

BELGISCHE VERENIGING VOOR SUIKERZIEKEN,
Godshuizenlaan 13, B-9000 GHENT.
Telephone (091) 25 94 59.

DENMARK

LANDSFORENINGEN FOR SUKKERSYGE,
St. Anna Plads 2, DK-5000 ODENSE.
Telephone (09) 12 90 06.

FINLAND

FINNISH DIABETES ASSOCIATION,
Diabeteskesus, SF-33680 TAMPERE 68.
Telephone 931-600 333.

FRANCE

ASSOCIATION FRANCAISE DES DIABETIQUES,
Boite Postale No. 101, F-75662 PARIS Cedex 14. (for visitors:
5 ter, rue d'Alesia, F-75014 PARIS).
Telephone 589 29 90.

GERMAN DEMOCRATIC REPUBLIC

GESELLSCHAFT FUER ENDOKRINOLOGIE UND
STOFFWECHSELKRANKHEITEN,
Sektion Diabetes, Zentralinstitut fuer Diabetes, DDR-2201
KARLSBURG.

GERMAN FEDERAL REPUBLIC

DEUTSCHER DIABETIKER-BUND e.V.,
Bahnhofstrass 74-76, D-4650 GELSENKIRCHEN.
Telephone 0209/15 080.

DEUTSCHE DIABETES-GESELLSCHAFT,
c/o Prof. Dr. K. D. Hepp, Staedt. Krankenhaus Muenchen-
Oberfoehring, Oberfoehringer Strasse 156, D-8000
MUENCHEN 81.

GREECE

HELLENIC DIABETOLOGIC ASSOCIATION,
4 Papadiamandopoulou Street, ATHENS 612.
Telephone 711-845.

HUNGARY

HUNGARIAN DIABETES ASSOCIATION,
Koranyi Sandor utca 2/a, H-1083 BUDAPEST VIII.

IRELAND

IRISH DIABETIC ASSOCIATION,
Ballyneety House, St. Laurence Road, Clontarf, DUBLIN 3.

ITALY

ASSOCIAZIONE ITALIANA PER LA DIFESA DEGLI
INTERESSI DIE DIABETICI,

Via del Scrofa 14, ROMA.
Telephone 65-43 784.

SOCIETA ITALIANA DI DIABETOLOGIA,
c/o Prof. G. M. Molinatti, Cattedra di Endocrinologia,
Corso Polonia 14, I-10126 TORINO.

LUXEMBOURG
ASSOCIATION LUXEMBOURGEOISE DU DIABETE,
B.P. 1316. LUXEMBOURG

MALTA
DIABETES ASSOCIATION,
P.O. Box 413 VALLETTA. Malta.

NETHERLANDS
DIABETES VERENIGING NEDERLAND,
Postbus 9210, 3506 GE UTRECHT. (for visitors:
Faustdreef 185, 3561 LG UTRECHT).
Telephone (030) 62 08 22.

NEDERLANDSE VERENIGING VOOR
DIABETESONDERZOEK,
c/o Dr. E. De Nobel (Secretary), Kliniek voor Inwendige
Ziekten, St. Radboud Ziekenhis, 6500 HB NIJMEGEN.

NORWAY
NORGES LANDSFORBUND FOR SUKKERSYKE,
Wdm. Thranes gt. 98, OSLO 1.

POLAND
SECTION FOR DIABETES,
Polish Association of Internal Medicine,
c/o Ul. Kopcinskiego 22, 91-738 LODZ.

PORTUGAL
ASSOCIACAO PROTECTORA DOS DIABETICOS DE
PORTUGAL,

Rua do Salitre 118/120, LISBON 2.
Telephone 68 00 41.

ROMANIA

UNION DES SOCIETIES DES SCIENCES MEDICALES,
DE LA REPUBLIQUE SOCIALISTE DE ROUMANIE,
8 rue Progresului, BUCHAREST.

SPAIN

SOCIEDAD ESPANOLA DE DIABETES,
Colegio Oficial de Medicos, Santa Isabel 51, MADRID 12.

SWEDEN

SVENSKA DIABETESFORBUNDET,
Box 266, S-101 23 STOCKHOLM. (for visitors: Vasagatan
38A STOCKHOLM).
Telephone (08) 23 66 25.

SWEDISH ENDOCRINE SOCIETY,
c/o Department of Endocrinology, Karolinska Hospital,
S-104 01 STOCKHOLM.

SWITZERLAND

SCHWEIZERISCHE DIABETES-GESELLSCHAFT,
(Association Suisse du Diabete) Stauffacherquai 36, CH-8004
ZURICH.
Telephone (01)-242 14 19.

TURKEY

TURK DIABET CEMIYETI,
Harbiye, Meyva Sokak 10, ISTANBUL.
Telephone 48 60 86.

UNITED KINGDOM

BRITISH DIABETIC ASSOCIATION,
10 Queen Anne Street, LONDON W1M 0BD.
Telephone (01)-323 1531.

YUGOSLAVIA
SAVEZ DRUSTAVA ZA ZASTITU OD DIJABETESA
JUGOSLAVIJE,
Krijesnice b.b., YU-41000 ZAGREB.
Telephone (041) 215 315.

REGION OF THE AMERICAS
NORTH AMERICA

CANADA
CANADIAN DIABETES ASSOCIATION,
78 Bond Street, TORONTO, Ontario M5B 2J8

L'ASSOCIATION DU DIABETE DU QUEBEC,
4565 de la Reine Marie, Suite 2223, MONTREAL,
Quebec H3W 1W5.
Telephone (514) 731-6406.

UNITED STATES
AMERICAN DIABETES ASSOCIATION,
2 Park Avenue, NEW YORK, N.Y. 10016.
Telephone (212) 683-7444.

CENTRAL AMERICA AND CARIBBEAN

BERMUDA
BERMUDA DIABETIC ASSOCIATION,
P.O. Box 1561, HAMILTON 5.
Telephone (809-29) 1-6365.

CUBA
SOCIEDAD CUBANA DE DIABETES,
Consejo Cientifico del MINSAP 23 y N, Vedado, HABANA 4.

DOMINICAN REPUBLIC
INSTITUTO NACIONAL DE ENDOCRINOLOGIA Y

NUTRITION, (INDEN).
Patronato Contra la Diabetes Inc., P.O. Box 1600,
SANTO DOMINGO.
Telephone 687-7033.

MEXICO
SOCIEDAD MEXICANA DE NUTRICION Y
ENDOCRINOLOGIA,
Vasca de Quiroga no. 15, Deleg. Tialpan,
1400 MEXICO D.F.

ASSOCIACION MEXICANA DE DIABETES A.C.,
Apartado Postal 52, Agencia de Correos "A", Garza
Garcia, N.L.

NETHERLANDS ANTILLES
DIABETIC ASSOCIATION OF CURACAO,
(SOKUDI).
P.O. Box 439, CURACAO.

PUERTO RICO
SOCIEDAD PUERTORRIQUENA DE
ENDOCRINOLOGIA Y DIABETOLOGIA,
c/o Dr. L. Haddock, Apartado 41174, Estacion Minillas,
SANTURCE. Puerto Rico 00940.

SOUTH AMERICA

ARGENTINA
SOCIEDAD ARGENTINA DE DIABETES,
Santa Fe 1171, BUENOS AIRES.

LIGA ARGENTINA DE PROTECCION AL
DIABETICO (LAPDI),
Tucuman 1584, BUENOS AIRES.
Telephone 40 81 85.

BRAZIL
SOCIEDADE BRASILEIRA DE DIABETES,
c/o Rua Moncorvo Filho 100, RIO DE JANEIRO—
CEP 20211.

ASSOCIACAO BRASILEIRA DE DIABETICOS,
Av. Paulista 2073, 21° Andar-Sala 2123, SAO PAULO—
CEP 01311.
Telephone 289-2941.

CHILE
SOCIEDAD CHILENA DE ENDOCRINOLOGIA Y
METABOLISMO,
Esmerelda 678, Casilla 23-D, SANTIAGO.

COLOMBIA
ASOCIACION COLOMBIANA DE DIABETES,
Avenida 39, No. 14-93, BOGOTA.
Telephone 245-43 50.

ECUADOR
ASOCIACION ECUATORIANA DE DIABETES,
c/o Hospital "Carlos Andrade Marin," Departamento
Medico del I.E.S.S. Servicio de Endocrinologia,
QUITO.

PARAGUAY
SOCIEDAD PARAGUAY DE DIABETOLOGIA,
c/o Circulo Paraguayo de Medicos, Luis A. Herrera 1588,
ASUNCION.

PERU
SOCIEDAD PERUANA DE ENDOCRINOLOGIA,
Casilla 435, LIMA.

SURINAME
STICHTING DIABETES SURINAME,

Gravenstraat 7 bov, PARAMARIBO.
Telephone 743-47.

URUGUAY
ASOCIACION DE DIABETICOS DEL URUGUAY,
Calle Paraquay 1273, MONTEVIDEO.
Telephone 91-62 14.

VENEZUELA
ASOCIACION VENEZOLANA DE DIABETES,
Av. Caracas 464, BARQUISIMETO.

SOCIEDAD VENEZOLANA DE ENDOCRINOLOGIA Y
METABOLISMO,
Apartado 61843, CARACAS 1041-A.

AFRICAN REGION

KENYA
KENYA DIABETIC ASSOCIATION,
P.O. Box 52951, NAIROBI,
Kenya.

MAURITIUS
THE MAURITIUS DIABETIC ASSOCIATION,
P.O. Box 17, ROSE HILL.

NIGERIA
DIABETES ASSOCIATION OF NIGERIA,
c/o Prof. T. O. Johnson (President), Department of Medicine,
College of Medicine, University of Lagos, P.M.B. 12003,
LAGOS.

SOUTH AFRICA
SOUTH AFRICAN DIABETES ASSOCIATION,
P.O. Box 32168, BRAAMFONTEIN 2017,

South Africa.
Telephone 39-6381.

SOCIETY FOR ENDOCRINOLOGY, METABOLISM
AND DIABETES OF SOUTHERN AFRICA,
c/o Dr. B. Joffe, 97 Clovelly Road, Greenside Extn.,
JOHANNESBURG 2193.

EASTERN MEDITERRANEAN REGION

CYPRUS
CYPRUS DIABETIC ASSOCIATION,
1 Kapota Street, PAPHOS.

EGYPT
EGYPTIAN SOCIETY FOR ENDOCRINOLOGY
METABOLISM AND DIABETES,
c/o Prof. N. Hashem, Paediatric Dept., Faculty
of Medicine, Ain-Shams University, 5 El-Goumhouria
Street, CAIRO.
Telephone 906-267.

IRAN
IRANIAN DIABETES SOCIETY,
P.O. Box 1646, TEHRAN.
Telephone 899921-24.

ISRAEL
ISRAEL DIABETES ASSOCIATION,
P.O. Box 432, JERUSALEM (for visitors: 72 Haneviim
Street, JERUSALEM).

PAKISTAN
THE DIABETIC ASSOCIATION OF PAKISTAN,
V-E/III, Main Mohammed Siddique Khan Trust Building,
Nazimabad, Paposhnagar, KARACHI.

SUDAN
SUDANESE DIABETIC ASSOCIATION,
P.O. Box 509, KHARTOUM.
Telephone 78 720.

TUNISIA
L'ASSOCIATION TUNISIENNE DES DIABETIQUES,
10 rue E. Nohelle, TUNIS.

SOUTH-EAST ASIAN REGION

BANGLADESH
DIABETIC ASSOCIATION OF BANGLADESH,
Shahbagh Avenue, DACCA 2.
Telephones 259 325—280 795.

INDIA
DIABETIC ASSOCIATION OF INDIA,
Maneckji Wadia Building, 1st Floor, Mahatma Gandhi Road,
BOMBAY 40 00 01.
Telephone 27 38 13.

SRI LANKA
DIABETIC ASSOCIATION OF SRI LANKA,
10 Trelawney Place, COLOMBO 4.

THAILAND
DIABETIC ASSOCIATION OF THAILAND,
Mongkutkao Hospital, Payatai, BANGKOK.

WESTERN PACIFIC REGION

AUSTRALIA
DIABETES FEDERATION OF AUSTRALIA,

c/o Mr. A. T. Harris (Secretary), 27 Brewer Street,
EAST PERTH, Western Australia 6000.

AUSTRALIAN DIABETES SOCIETY,
c/o Dr. G. B. Senator (Secretary),
Department of Endocrinology, Royal Hobart Hospital,
G.P.O. Box 1061 L, HOBART, Tasmania 7001.

FIJI
FIJI DIABETIC ASSOCIATION,
P.O. Box 775, SUVA.

JAPAN
JAPAN DIABETIC SOCIETY,
3-38-11 Hongo Sky Building, Room 403, Hongo,
Bunkyo-ku, TOKYO 113.

NEW ZEALAND
DIABETIC ASSOCIATION OF NEW ZEALAND,
P.O. Box 3656, WELLINGTON.

PHILIPPINES
PHILIPPINE DIABETES ASSOCIATION,
Room 352, Medical Center Manila, MANILA.

REPUBLIC OF KOREA
KOREAN DIABETES ASSOCIATION,
c/o Dept. of Internal Medicine, Seoul National University
Hospital, 28 Yeongun-Dong Chongro-ku, SEOUL 110.

SINGAPORE
DIABETIC SOCIETY OF SINGAPORE,
Kelliney Road, P.O. Box 82, SINGAPORE 9123.

Appendix F

USEFUL PHRASES
IN FOREIGN LANGUAGES

These translations were provided by the consular offices of the countries in question, or, if they failed to respond, by college foreign-language professors.

Danish

I am a diabetic.
Jeg lider af sukkersyge.

Call a doctor, please.
Vær venlig at få fat i en læge.

Quick! Some orange juice or a Coca-Cola, please. I am (he is, she is) a diabetic. I am (he is, she is) having an insulin reaction.
Hurtigt! Venligst skaf noget appelsinsaft eller en coca cola. Jeg (han, hun) lider af sukkersyge. Jeg har (han har, hun har) fået et insulinchok.

Do you have some fruit and cheese for dessert?
Har De noget frugt eller ost til dessert?

Does this have sugar in it? I am diabetic and cannot eat anything with sugar in it.
Indeholder dette sukker? Jeg lider af sukkersyge og kan ikke spise noget, der indeholder sukker.

No, thank you. I am on a strict diet and cannot eat that.
Nej tak. Jeg er på streng diæt og kan ikke spise det.

Dutch (Belangrijk)

I am a diabetic.
Ik ben een diabeticus.

217

Call a doctor, please.
Roep alsjeblieft een dokter.

Quick! Some orange juice or a Coca-Cola, please. I am (he is, she is) a diabetic. I am (he is, she is) having an insulin reaction.
Vlug! Geef mij alsjeblieft wat sinaasappelsap of een Coca-Cola. Ik ben (hij is, zij is) een diabeticus. Ik val (hij valt, zij valt) anders flauw.

Do you have some fruit and cheese for dessert?
Hebt U ook fruit en kaas voor desert?

Does this have sugar in it? I am diabetic and cannot eat anything with sugar in it.
Zit her suiker in? Ik ben een diabeticus en mag niets eten waar suiker in zit.

No, thank you. I am on a strict diet and cannot eat that.
Neen, dank U. Ik ben op een streng diëet en mag dat niet eten.

Finnish

I am a diabetic.
Olen sokeritautinen.

Call a doctor, please.
Kutsukaa lääkäri, olkaa hyvä.

Quick! Some orange juice or a Coca-Cola, please. I am (he is, she is) a diabetic. I am (he is, she is) having an insulin reaction.
Nopeasti! Appelsiinimehua tai coca-colaa, olkaa hyvä. Olen (hän on) sokeritautinen. Minulla on insuliinireaktio.

Do you have some fruit and cheese for dessert?
Onko teillä hedelmiä ja juustoa jälkiruoaksi?

Does this have sugar in it? I am diabetic and cannot eat anything with sugar in it.
Onko tässä sokeria? Olen sokeritautinen enkä voi syödä mitään, jossa on sokeria.

No, thank you. I am on a strict diet and cannot eat that.
Ei kiitos. Olen tiukalla ruokavaliolla enkä voi syödä sitä.

French

I am a diabetic.
Je suis diabétique.

Call a doctor, please.
Allez chercher un médecin, s'il vous plaît.

Quick! Some orange juice or a Coca-Cola, please. I am (he is, she is) a diabetic. I am (he is, she is) having an insulin reaction.
Vite! Du jus d'orange ou un Coca-Cola, je vous en prie. Je suis (il est, elle est) diabétique, et j'ai (il a, elle a) la malaise d'insuline.

Do you have some fruit and cheese for dessert?
Avez-vous des fruits et du fromage pour dessert?

Does this have sugar in it? I am diabetic and cannot eat anything with sugar in it.
Est-ce que ceci contient du sucre? Je suis diabétique et je ne peux rien manger que contienne du sucre.

No, thank you. I am on a strict diet and cannot eat that.
Non, merci. Je dois suivre un régime rigoureux, et je ne peux pas manger cela.

German

I am a diabetic.
Ich bin zuckerkrank.

Call a doctor, please.
Rufen Sie bitte einen Arzt.

Quick! Some orange juice or a Coca-Cola, please. I am (he is, she is) a diabetic. I am (he is, she is) having an insulin reaction.
Schnell! Bitte etwas Orangensaft oder Coca-Cola. Ich bin (er ist, sie ist) zuckerkrank. Die Insulinspritze wirkt augenblicklich.

Do you have some fruit and cheese for dessert?
Haben Sie etwas Früchte und Käse zum Nachtisch?

Does this have sugar in it? I am diabetic and cannot eat anything with sugar in it.
Enthält dies Zucker? Ich bin zuckerkrank und darf nichts essen, was Zucker enthält.

No, thank you. I am on a strict diet and cannot eat that.
Nein, danke schön. Ich muss strenge Diät einhalten und darf das nicht essen.

Greek

I am a diabetic.
Eimai diaviticos.

Call a doctor, please.
Paracalo calesete yiatro.

Quick! Some orange juice or a Coca-Cola, please. I am (he is, she is) a diabetic. I am (he is, she is) having an insulin reaction.
Grigora Paracalo ligi portocalada ei koka-kola eimai (einai) diaviticos eho (ehei) andidrasi insoulinis.

Do you have some fruit and cheese for dessert?
Ehete frouta kae tyri dia epidorpion?

Does this have sugar in it? I am diabetic and cannot eat anything with sugar in it.
Afto periehei zahari? Eimal diaviticos kae den epitrepetae tipotae glyco.

No, thank you. I am on a strict diet and cannot eat that.
Ohi efharisto. Kano afstiri diaita kae den mporo na to trogo.

Italian

I am a diabetic.
Io sono diabetico.

Call a doctor, please.
Per favore chiami un dottore.

Quick! Some orange juice or a Coca-Cola, please. I am (he is, she is) a diabetic. I am (he is, she is) having an insulin reaction.

Portatemi subito dell'aranciata o del Coca-Cola. Io sono (egli è, ella è) diabetico. Sono (egli è; ella è) sotto l'effetto dell'insulina.

Do you have some fruit and cheese for dessert?
Avete della frutta o formaggio?

Does this have sugar in it? I am diabetic and cannot eat anything with sugar in it.
Contiene zucchero? Io sono diabetico e lo zucchero mi nuoce.

No, thank you. I am on a strict diet and cannot eat that.
No, grazie. Io sono sotto rigorosa cura e non posso mangiare questo.

Japanese

I am a diabetic.
Watakushi wa tōnȳobȳo-kanja desu.

Call a doctor, please.
Isha o yondekudasai.

Quick! Some orange juice or a Coca-Cola, please. I am (he is, she is) a diabetic. I am (he is, she is) having an insulin reaction.
Suguni! Orenji-jusu ka Koka-Kora o kudasai. Watakushi wa (kare wa, kanopo wa) tōnȳobȳo-kanja desu. Watakushi wa (kare wa, kanojo wa) inshurin han nochu desu.

Do you have some fruit and cheese for dessert?
Dezāto ni kudamono ka chizu ga arimasuka.

Does this have sugar in it? I am diabetic and cannot eat anything with sugar in it.
Koreni wa sato ga haitte imasuka. Watakushi wa tōnȳobȳo-kanja de sato no haitteiru mono wa nani mo taberaremasen.

No, thank you. I am on a strict diet and cannot eat that.
Iie, kekko desu. Watakushi wa shokuji-ryohochu desunode sore wa taberaremasen.

Norwegian

I am a diabetic.
Jeg har sukkersyke.

Call a doctor, please.
Vær så snild og tilkall en lege.

Quick! Some orange juice or a Coca-Cola, please. I am (he is, she is) a diabetic. I am (he is, she is) having an insulin reaction.
Fort! Gi meg litt appelsinsaft eller Coca-Cola er De snild. Jeg har (han har, hun har) sukkersyke. Jeg har (han har, hun har) insulin-reaksjon.

Do you have some fruit and cheese for dessert?
Har De noe frukt eller ost til dessert?

Does this have sugar in it? I am diabetic and cannot eat anything with sugar in it.
Er det sukker i dette? Jeg har sukkersyke og kan ikke spise noe som har sukker.

No, thank you. I am on a strict diet and cannot eat that.
Nei takk. Jeg er på streng diett og kan ikke spise dette.

Portuguese

I am a diabetic.
Eu sou diabético.

Call a doctor, please.
Chame um médico, por favor.

Quick! Some orange juice or a Coca-Cola, please. I am (he is, she is) a diabetic. I am (he is, she is) having an insulin reaction.
Depressa! Um suco de laranja ou uma coca-cola, por favor. Eu sou (êle é, ela é) diabético. Estou (êle está, ela está) tendo una reação de insulina.

Do you have some fruit and cheese for dessert?
O senhor (a senhora) tem alguma fruta ou queijo para a sobremesa?

Does this have sugar in it? I am diabetic and cannot eat anything with sugar in it.
Iso contém açucar? Eu sou diabético e não posso comer nada que contenha açucar.

No, thank you. I am on a strict diet and cannot eat that.
Não, obrigado. Eu estou numa dieta rigorosa e não posso comer isto.

Russian

I am a diabetic.
Ya diabetic.

Call a doctor, please.
Vysovite, pazhahlasta, doctora.

Quick! Some orange juice or a Coca-Cola, please. I am (he is, she is) a diabetic. I am (he is, she is) having an insulin reaction.
Bystro! Pazhahlusta, sok ili koka-kola. Ya (on, ona) diabetic. U menya (u nego, u nee) insulinovaya reaktzia.

Do you have some fruit and cheese for dessert?
Yest li u vas fructi ili syr na desert?

Does this have sugar in it? I am diabetic and cannot eat anything with sugar in it.
Yest li v etom sakhar? Ya diabetic i ne mogu yest nichevo s sakharom.

No, thank you. I am on a strict diet and cannot eat that.
Nyet, spasibo. Ya na strogoi diete i ne mogu yest etovo.

Spanish

I am a diabetic.
Soy diabético.

Call a doctor, please.
Favor de llamar al médico.

Quick! Some orange juice or a Coca-Cola, please. I am (he is, she is) a diabetic. I am (he is, she is) having an insulin reaction.
¡Aprisa! Un vaso de jugo de naranjo o una Coca-Cola por favor. Soy diabético (él es diabético, ella es diabética). Me (le, le) está dando una reacción insulínica.

Do you have some fruit and cheese for dessert?
¿Hay fruta y queso de postre?

Does this have sugar in it? I am diabetic and cannot eat anything with sugar in it.
¿Hay azúcar en esto? Soy diabético y no puedo comer nada que contenga azúcar.

No, thank you. I am on a strict diet and cannot eat that.
No, gracias. Estoy a dieta rigurosa y no puedo comer eso.

Swedish

I am a diabetic.
Jag är sockersjuk.

Call a doctor, please.
Var snäll och kalla på en doktor.

Quick! Some orange juice or a Coca-Cola, please. I am (he is, she is) a diabetic. I am (he is, she is) having an insulin reaction.
Skynda er! Lite apelsinsaft eller en Coca-Cola, är ni snäll. Jag är (han är, hon är) sockersjuk. Jag (han, hon) fått ett insulinanfall.

Do you have some fruit and cheese for dessert?
Har ni lite frukt och ost till efterrätt?

Does this have sugar in it? I am diabetic and cannot eat anything with sugar in it.
Innehåller detta socker? Jag är sockersjuk och kan inte äta något som innehåller socker.

No, thank you. I am on a strict diet and cannot eat that.
Nej tack. Jag håller sträng diet och kan inte äta det.

DIABETIC IDENTIFICATION CARD IN FOREIGN LANGUAGES

The text of this message is "The bearer of this card is diabetic and is taking insulin injections. In case of sudden confusion or weakness, please give him two tablespoonfuls of sugar in water, and send for a doctor immediately."

The translations for Danish, Dutch (Belangrijk), French, German, Italian, Norwegian, Portuguese, and Spanish were supplied by the British Diabetic Association. All others were obtained from consular offices of the country in question.

Each of these identification cards is designed to facilitate removal from the book.

. . . .

Danish

INDEHAVEREN AF DETTE KORT ER DIABETIKER OG INDTAGER INSULIN. I TILFAELDE AF ET PLUDSELIGT ILDEBEFINDENDE ELLER BEVIDSTLØSHED BØR MAN LADE PATIENTEN DRIKKE 2 SPISESKEFULDE SUKKER OPLØST I VAND, OG DEN NAERMESTE LAEGE BØR OMGAENDE TILKALDES.

Dutch (*Belangrijk*)

DE DRAGER VAN DEZE KAART IS SUIKERPATIENT EN
GEBRUIKT INSULINE. IN GEVAL VAN PLOTSELINGE
VERWARRING OF FLAUWTE GEEFT A.U.B. TWEE
VOLLE EETLEPELS SUIKER IN WATER EN HAAL DE
DICHTSTBIJZIJNDE DOKTER.

Finnish

TÄMÄN KORTIN HALTIJA SAIRASTAA SOKERITAUTIA
JA OTTAA INSULIINI PRUISKEITA. ÄKILLISEN HÄIRIÖ-
TAI HEIKKOUSTILAN SATTUESSA, ANNA HÄNELLE
KAKSI RUOKALUSIKALLISTA SOKERIA VETEEN SEKOIT-
ETTUNA JA KUTSU VÄLITTÖMÄSTI LÄÄKÄRI PAIKALLE.

French

LE PORTEUR DE CETTE CARTE EST DIABÉTIQUE ET EN
RÉGIME D'INSULINE. EN CAS DE PERTURBATION OÙ
DÉ DEFAILLANCE SUBITES, PRIÈRE DE FAIRE PRENDRE
DEUX CUILLERÉES À SOUPE DE SUCRE DISSOUS DANS
DE L'EAU ET DE FAIRE VENIR TOUT DE SUITE UN
MÉDECIN.

. . . .

German

DER TRÄGER DIESER KARTE HAT ZUCKERKRANKHEIT
UND NIMMT INSULIN. IM FALLE DER UNERWARTETE
VERWIRRUNG ODER OHNMACHT, ZWEI ESSLÖFFEL
ZUCKER IM WASSER SOLL GEGEBEN WERDEN. BITTE
VERSTANDIGEN SIE SOFORT EINEN ARZT.

Greek

Ο ΦΕΡΩΝ ΤΗΝ ΚΑΡΤΑΝ ΑΥΤΗΝ ΕΙΝΑΙ ΔΙΑΒΗΤΙΚΟΣ ΚΑΙ ΤΟΥ ΚΑΝΟΥΝ ΕΝΕΣΕΙΣ ΙΝΣΟΥΛΙΝΗΣ. ΕΙΣ ΠΕΡΙΠΤΩΣΙΝ ΞΑΦΝΙΚΗΣ ΣΥΓΧΙΣΕΩΣ Η ΑΔΥΝΑΜΙΑΣ, ΠΑΡΑΚΑΛΕΙΣΘΕ ΟΠΩΣ ΤΟΥ ΔΩΣΗΤΕ ΔΥΟ ΚΟΥΤΑΛΙΕΣ ΤΗΣ ΣΟΥΠΑΣ ΣΑΚΧΑ-ΡΕΩΣ ΕΝΤΟΣ ΥΔΑΤΟΣ ΚΑΙ ΚΑΛΕΣΗΤΕ ΑΜΕΣΩΣ ΙΑΤΡΟΝ.

. . . .

Italian

IL PORTATORE DI QUESTA CARTA E DIABETICO E SI INIETTA INSULIN. SE IN CASO DI MALATTIA SUBI-TANEA, SI PREGA DI DARLE 2 CUCCHIAI PIENI DI ZUCCHERO IN ACQUA E FAR VENIRE SUBITO UN DOTTORE.

Japanese

このカードの所持者は糖尿病患者でインシュリン療養中です。 突然発作が起きましたらスプーン2匙の砂糖を水に加え飲ませて下さい。 そして直ちに医者を呼んで下さい。

Norwegian

JEG HAR SUKKERSYKE. HVIS JEG ER BEVISTLØS, ELLER OPPFØRER MEG UNORMALT, KAN DET VAERE AT JEG HAR INSULINFØLING ELLER INSULINSJOKK. HVIS JEG KAN SVELGE, GI MEG SUKKER, SJOKOLADE, FRUKST-SAFT ELLER EN SØTET DRIKK. HVIS JEG IKKE KLARER A SVELGE, ELLER HVIS JEG IKKE KOMMER MEG SNART, VAER SÅ SNILD A FA TAK I EN LEGE ELLER SEND MEG TIL ET SYKEHUS.

Portuguese

O PORTADOR DESTE CARTAO É DIABÉTICO E INJECTA INSULINA. SE FOR ENCONTRADO ACIDENTALMENTE EM ESTADO DE CONFUSAO OU DE FRAQUEZA, É FAVOR FAZÊ-LO INGERIR AGUA COM 2 COLHERES DE SOPA DE AÇUCAR E CONDUZI-LO RAPIDAMENTE AO MEDICO MAIS PRÓXIMO.

. . . .

Russian

ПРЕДЪЯВИТЕЛЬ ЭТОЙ КАРТОЧКИ — ДИАБЕТИК И ПОЛУЧАЕТ ИНЪЕКЦИИ ИНСУЛИНА. В СЛУЧАЕ ВНЕЗАПНОГО ЗАМЕША-ТЕЛЬСТВА ИЛИ СЛАБОСТИ, ПОЖАЛУЙСТА, ДАЙТЕ ЕМУ ДВЕ СТОЛОВЫХ ЛОЖКИ САХАРУ В ВОДЕ И ОТПРАВЛЯЙТЕ ЕГО НЕМЕДЛЕННО К ДОКТОРУ.

Spanish

ME INYECTO INSULINA. SOY DIABÉTICO. SI ME ENCUENTRA DESMAYADO DÉME DOS CUCHARADAS DE AZÚCAR EN LÍQUIDO Y SÍRVASE VD. COMUNICAR CON EL MÉDICO O EL HOSPITAL MÁS CERCANO.

. . . .

Swedish

INNEHAVAREN AV DETTA KORT ÄR`SOCKERSJUK OCH TAR INSULININSPRUTNINGAR. OM HAN PLÖTSLIGT VISAR TECKEN PÅ FÖRVIRRING ELLER SVAGHET, VAR VÄNLIG GIV HONOM TVÅ TESKEDAR SOCKER I VATTEN OCH SKICKA EFTER EN LÄKARE OMEDELBART.

Appendix H

THE GUTHRIES ON TESTING

Diana Guthrie, R.N., Ed.S., F.A.A.N., C., and Richard Guthrie, M.D.

We have been, for many years, internationally known for maintaining "tight control" of blood-glucose levels in children having diabetes—that is, managing their diabetes so that they had normal, or near normal, blood-glucose levels the majority of the time. We believe this should be done without the occurrence of significant insulin reactions. For many years we had no facilities for home blood-glucose testing, so management had to be done with urine testing alone. Normal, functioning adults with long-term diabetes and no vascular disease proved it could be done with urine testing alone if the urine testing was properly done and properly interpreted. Later we documented the good control with glycosylated hemoglobin (the two- to three-month average blood-glucose level) values in or near the normal range. Then came the blood-glucose monitor, which allowed the individual and family members, as well as the professionals, to have an even better idea as to the blood-sugar level. All of these are now tools we can use to ensure the best possible control. None should be ignored, as each gives a different piece of information.

Yes, we recommend blood-glucose monitoring as the most accurate way now available of determining control levels, and it is right, as a parent of a small child, to want to have the security of knowing that the bedtime blood test is at a "safe" level. Remember, however, that blood-glucose levels are a dynamic, constantly changing phenomenon and that a blood test registers only a point or moment in time. It is a very important test, but all confidence should not be placed in one test alone. A blood-sugar level at bedtime could be quite normal and yet at 3:00 A.M. or 10:00 A.M. or 2:00 P.M. be quite high or low. Both glycosylated hemoglobin (Hgb A_1C or Hgb

239

A_1) and first-voided urine tests—especially in children in whom renal thresholds (the points at which the kidney allows glucose to be passed from the body into the urine) are lower than "average"— give information over a period of time, and properly used can give more information than a momentary blood sugar. It is true that most children do not mind the blood test, but some do. For those children whose control is relatively stable and the glycosylated hemoglobin test is normal or near normal, indicating good control, urine testing can be routinely used with blood testing used intermittently, especially for suspected hypoglycemia or as a reassurance at bedtime. Urine testing should always be used when the child is ill or if there is any doubt in the wildly fluctuating blood-glucose levels. In both these instances, blood-glucose testing combined with urine testing especially for ketones should be used.

Most of all, be both knowledgeable of and flexible to the child's response to his or her disease. Keep these goals in mind: twenty-four-hour distributed insulin coverage for normalized blood-glucose levels, flexibility of lifestyle, and ability of the child (and adult) to participate, cooperate, and/or adapt to the diabetes management program.

1. For children under school age in whom hypoglycemia is harder to detect than in older children and in whom it has greater consequences, blood testing should be routine, with concurrent urine testing for ketones in illness or consistently high blood sugar and frequent blood testing when hypoglycemia is suspected. Overall control should be checked by a first-voided urine test two or three times a week.

2. For children from school age (five to six years) to adolescence—where hypoglycemia is easier to detect, consequences of hypoglycemia are not as great, renal threshold is low (reflecting blood-glucose levels reasonably well, and control is good as documented by Hgb A_1C levels)—encourage blood-glucose testing. Alternate with urine testing using two-drop Clinitest on first-voided specimen before meals and at bedtime with concurrent blood testing in illness and when hypoglycemia is suspected.

3. All others use blood testing as a routine with concurrent urine testing for ketones in illness.
4. Remember that a second-voided urine test reflects blood sugar one-half to one hour before the urine specimen is taken and tested; a first-voided test represents blood sugar collected in the urine over a longer period.

INDEX

243

Holland
  diabetic identification card, 227
  meals, 99
  useful phrases in, 217–218
Hospital, diabetics in the, 136–140
How to Live with Diabetes (Dolger
    and Seeman), 31, 72–73
Hungarian Diabetes Association,
    207
Hunter, Beatrice Trum, 160
Hyperglycemia, 142
Hypoglycemia, 142, 149, 150, 240
Hypoglycemic twinges, 13

Ice cream, 159, 160
Identification cards, 97, 225–237
  Danish, 225
  Dutch, 227
  Finnish, 227
  French, 229
  German, 229
  Greek, 231
  Italian, 231
  Japanese, 233
  Norwegian, 233
  Portuguese, 235
  Russian, 235
  Spanish, 237
  Swedish, 237
Indian cuisine, 59
Instituto Nacional de
    Endocrinologia y Nutrition,
    211
Insulin, 17–20, 103
  changing injection sites, 134–135
  discovery of, 8
  freezing of, 94
  giving injections of, 114–116
  human, 149
  infusion pumps, 148–149
  prescription requirements for, 25

schedule, 148–149
synthetic, 149
traveling abroad with, 93–94
Insulin shock, 13, 35, 68
  glucagon for, 115
  recognizing symptoms of,
    107–114
Intermedic, 96–97, 203
International Association for
    Medical Assistance to
    Travelers, 202–203
International Diabetes Federation,
    206–216
International Health Care Service,
    203
International SOS Assistance,
    203–204
Iranian Diabetes Society, 214
Irish Diabetic Association, 207
Israel Diabetes Association, 214
Italian
  cuisine, 56, 157
  diabetic identification card, 231
  meals, 98, 99
  useful phrases in, 220–221
Italian Diabetic Association,
    207–208

Japan Diabetic Society, 216
Japanese
  diabetic identification card,
    233
  meals, 100
  useful phrases in, 221
Jaqua, Ida, 38
Jenkins, Dr. David, 157, 159
Jet lag, 90–93, 167–169
Johnson, Dr. Samuel, 76
Johnson and Johnson Company,
    20
Jones, Jeanne, 176